Keys to the
Medical Front Office

Second Edition

This book is designed as an informational guide and is not to be used as a clinical or legal reference. It is published as a general resource only and sold with the understanding that the publisher is not engaged in rendering medical care or legal advice. The contents are not intended for diagnosis and treatment of an illness, or as a substitute for legal counsel. Always consult your doctor, medical expert, or attorney.

Copyright © 2013 Anne Seymour Johnson
Johnson Key Elements
ISBN: 0984539514
ISBN-13: 978-0984539512
LCCN: 2012949777
Printed in the United States of America

To my Mother,
For instilling in me a love of books
and thirst for knowledge

CONTENTS

Preface

As a former medical office manager, there never seemed to be enough time to properly welcome and on-board new employees. My efforts to train and orient new hires were haphazard at best, and for more times than I would like to admit, their first days on the job were often baptism by fire.

The health care organization I was working for provided an excellent company-wide orientation, introducing new employees to its mission statement, values, policies, and benefits package. The presentation addressed the compulsory health, legal, safety, and compliance issues, and painted an excellent view of the company culture. It laid the foundation; my responsibility was to build upon it with an equally structured and informative, site-specific session.

The reality was, however, that my orientations usually consisted of a courtesy meeting where I handed the new employee a half dozen pages of "useful information," gave the requisite office tour, and made a quick introduction to the staff member they would be shadowing. I was lucky to have dedicated and hard-working employees to readily assist with this task, but they were often pulled from the assignment because of office demands, and the new hire was suddenly left in the hot seat in front of a ringing phone. They all survived, of course, but having to sink or swim, is obviously not good for productivity or morale.

A self-proclaimed visionary, I desperately wanted to develop and implement an educational and organized on-boarding program, and arm new staff members with an arsenal of resources, which would include an "everything you need to know about the office" handbook I wanted to put together. I envisioned a comprehensive guide filled with a wealth of practical information that would serve to:

- Promote a positive first impression by showing new employees they are valued and supported
- Equip them with the tools they would need to confidently and effectively perform their job duties
- Establish consistency and structure for orientations of future hires

But I never had the time.

When my mother was no longer able to live on her own due to the progression of Alzheimer's disease, I resigned from my position to become her full-time caregiver. During this time, I had the opportunity to research and write the guide I always wanted to produce, *Keys to the Medical Front Office.*

Introduction

The health care industry continues to hire at an alarming rate and remains a bright spot in an otherwise bleak labor market. Despite economic times, the demand for health care workers is on the rise and shows no signs slowing down.

CLASSIFIED

Medical Front Office

Busy multi-physician practice seeks enthusiastic and organized individual with professional demeanor and exceptional customer service skills to join our team.

Experienced preferred but will train the right person
(555) 555-2222

Keys to the Medical Front Office is an essential resource for:

- Anyone interested in entering the high-demand field of health care
- Job applicants who want to impress employers with their knowledge and problem solving ability
- Current health care employees looking to develop core competencies for future promotional opportunities
- Medical office managers who need support and structure with new employee training and orientation

Written in outline form, incorporating a just-the-facts format, *Keys to the Medical Front Office* quickly introduces you to the key elements of the medical front office, and starts you on your career as a customer service employee in the exciting and fast-growing field of health care.

Part I

Customer Service

Patients come into the medical office for a variety of reasons:

- New patient appointments
- Routine checkups
- Follow-up visits
- Illness or injury
- Health management
- Patient education
- Questions concerning their plan of care
- Completion of paperwork

Simply, they have a problem or concern and need assistance.

Providing assistance is the role of the front office staff. Front office employees must have the personality and composure to work in a demanding, fast-paced environment. Superior customer service skills are essential.

- Greet and register patients
- Schedule appointments
- Answer telephones and record messages
- Collect co-payments
- Prepare referrals
- Verify insurance eligibility
- Manage medical records
- Organize and distribute mail
- Enter patient charges into database
- Explain practice policies and procedures to patients
- Maintain waiting room area

Accomplishing these tasks can be difficult when several people require your attention at the same time:

- Telephone is ringing
- Patient is waiting to be registered
- Courier needs a signature for a delivery
- Provider has a question about the schedule

How do you handle multiple people simultaneously while demonstrating excellent customer service?

Acknowledgement

Most people do not mind waiting a minute when they see you are busy, but they usually will not remain calm without an acknowledgement. Acknowledgement can be as simple as obtaining eye contact, smiling, a pleasant nod of your head, and "Thank you for your patience; I will be with you in a moment." Greeting patients acknowledges their presence, makes them feel welcomed, and shows you value their time.

Whenever possible address patients by name. Commit to it. Calling people by their name makes them feel important and appreciated. It is helpful to introduce yourself first, as it can be uncomfortable for the patient when you call them by name, but they do not yet know your name. Doing so instantly establishes a personal rapport.

Use discretion in how you address someone. Some people prefer to be addressed casually by their first name, while others prefer to be addressed formally by their title.

CUSTOMER SERVICE 5/10 RULE

- Think of the area 10 feet around you as your personal service zone
- Make eye contact with others at ten feet
- Greet them at five feet
- Smile, smile, smile

THE ART OF LISTENING

Listening is an active art, not a passive one. It is the conscious effort to hear the words the other person is saying and to try to interpret, comprehend, and respond.

- Be fully present in the moment
- Give your undivided attention
- Concentrate on what is being said
- Visualize what the other person is saying
- Try not to anticipate what he or she is about to say
- Listen without interruption
- Repeat what was said to show you listened and understood

THE SIGNIFICANCE OF BODY LANGUAGE

Body language is the silent form of communication. It includes posture, facial expressions, gestures, proximity, and much more. Some professionals estimate that body language makes up for as much as 90 percent of all communication, while the spoken word is responsible for only about 10 percent.

Eye Contact:	Obtaining and maintaining eye contact shows acknowledgement and interest.
Facial Expression:	A pleasant facial expression and smile convey warmth and a caring attitude.
Posture:	Good posture communicates professionalism and confidence. Facing toward the other person shows genuine interest in what he or she is saying.
Proximity:	Create a comfortable amount of personal space between yourself and others. Avoid getting too close or being too far away.

DEALING WITH DIFFICULT PEOPLE

This type of situation requires tact and self-control. Do not lose your patience or composure. Remaining calm and listening can prevent an unpleasant situation from escalating.

- Listen through to the end of the story
- Avoid trigger words and phrases that can cause people to become more difficult:
    - "Please calm down"
    - "I want you to...."
    - "You have to...."
- View the situation from the other person's perspective
- Don't take it personally
- Never let personal pride or prejudice become a factor
- Try not to interrupt
- Maintain eye contact
- Empathize with their situation
- Validate their feelings

  Deal with their feelings, and then deal with the problem.

- Remain focused on the problem
- Ask questions for clarification and to obtain more information
- Verify what took place and ask how the situation can be resolved
- Offer a solution
- Mutually agree to the solution
- Follow up to make sure the patient was satisfied with the resolution

Be proactive, not reactive. Patients will feel validated knowing their concerns are being heard and addressed. Listening, showing empathy, and offering a solution have considerable impact in helping to diffuse a difficult situation.

Make your customer service legendary. The number one reason a person stops patronizing a business is poor customer service. Providing superior service must be the priority. Patients demand it. Employees who exemplify unsurpassed customer service possess the following traits:

- Communication skills
- Critical thinking skills
- Empathy
- Enthusiasm
- Initiative
- Knowledge
- Listening skills
- Optimism
- Problem-solving skills
- Professionalism
- Resilience
- Upbeat personality

A customer is the most important visitor on our premises.
He is not dependent on us. We are dependent on him.
He is not an interruption in our work.
He is the purpose of it.
He is not an outsider in our business. He is part of it.
We are not doing him a favor by serving him.
He is doing us a favor by giving us the opportunity to do so.

Mahatma Gandhi

MY KEY NOTES

Part II

Patient Rights, Privacy & HIPAA

Congress enacted HIPAA, Health Insurance Portability and Accountably Act, in 1996. It is a comprehensive federal law that protects and safeguards the privacy of an individual's protected health information. The Department of Health and Human Services is responsible for creating the regulations, and the Office of Civil Rights is responsible for its enforcement. HIPAA is a mandatory federal law. There are penalties for failure to comply. HIPAA:

- Creates standards to protect the privacy and security of patients' protected health information (PHI)
- Grants the right of patients to access and amend their PHI
- Establishes National Provider Identifiers (NPI)
- Holds violators accountable if patient rights and privacy are compromised
- Combats waste, fraud, and abuse in health insurance
- Standardizes fee schedules and billing
- Reduces administrative costs
- Institutes the right of individuals to maintain health insurance when they move from one job to another

PATIENT RIGHTS, PRIVACY & HIPAA

Key Terms

Authorization
To give permission or grant power to

Confidentiality
Preserving the legal right to privacy of an individual's PHI

Consent
Permission, agreement

Covered Entity
- Providers who submits bills electronically
- Health care plans
- Health care clearinghouses

Disclosure
Providing, releasing, or transferring access of an individual's PHI to anyone outside the immediate covered entity

Expressed Consent
- Oral: Permission expressed through speech
- Written: Permission conveyed through documentation

Fee Schedule
List of services and corresponding charges

HIPAA Privacy Rule
Part of HIPAA law that addresses accessing, saving, and sharing of protected health information

HIPAA Security Rule
Part of HIPAA law that addresses the standards established to protect the creation, maintenance, and transmission of protected health information

Implied Consent
Permission inferred from an individual's behavior or silence

Informed Consent
Signed, witnessed, and dated permission to a covered entity

Minimum Necessary Standard
Access to PHI should be limited to only what you need to know to perform your job duties

National Payer Identifier

Unique identification number, mandated by HIPAA, assigned to entities involved in the claims payment process; also known as the Health Plan ID

Notice Of Privacy Practices (NPP)

Document required by HIPAA that providers must issue to patients on the first day of service. It describes how the practice manages, uses, and shares your PHI.

National Provider Identifier (NPI)

Unique ten-digit number, mandated by HIPAA, used to identify health care providers

Privacy

Individual's right to decide what information he or she wants disclosed

Protected Health Information (PHI)

HIPAA regulations define PHI as any spoken, written, or electronic information that relates to past, present, and future physical or mental health conditions of the patient including:

- Name
- Address
- Phone number
- Date of birth
- Social security number
- Fax number
- URL address
- Medical record (past, present, and future plan of care)
  - *When* treatment was provided
  - *What* treatment was provided
  - *Where* treatment was provided
  - *Why* treatment was provided
  - *Who* provided the treatment
- Account numbers
- Advance directive
- Insurance information
- Vehicle and serial numbers
- Fingerprints
- Full face photo

NOTICE OF PRIVACY PRACTICES FORM:

NOTICE OF PRIVACY PRACTICES
Health Park Family Medicine Center

This notice contains important information about your
Protected Health Information (PHI).
Please review it carefully.

Uses and Disclosures

Treatment

Protected Health Information may be used by staff members or released to other health care professionals for evaluating your health, diagnosing medical conditions, and providing treatment.

Payment

PHI may be used to obtain payment from your insurance plan or other sources of coverage such as Workers' Compensation or an automobile insurer in the event of a motor vehicle accident.

Law Enforcement Purposes

PHI may be released to law enforcement agencies to facilitate investigations or to comply with mandated government reporting.

Public Health & Safety

The law requires reporting of certain communicable diseases to the state Department of Health.

Office Administration

PHI may be used to support budgeting, financial reporting, and other activities that affect and evaluate quality.

Other Purposes and Disclosures

- Disclosure of your PHI for any reason other than listed above requires a written authorization.
- You have a right to inspect, copy, and amend your Protected Health Information.
- You have a right to a list of all disclosures.
- If you feel your privacy protections have been violated, you have a right to file a complaint. Please direct any questions or concerns to our Privacy Officer: John Bell (555) 555-3333.

Patient Signature:

Date:

WHAT:	**PATIENT RIGHTS**
WHY:	**Right to privacy**
	Informed consent

Patients are entitled to certain rights when they receive medical care:

- Right to respect, courtesy, and dignity
- Right to autonomy: Independent decision making
- Right to informed consent
- Right to confidentiality and privacy of protected health information (PHI):
  - PHI includes personal, medical, and financial information
  - Patients have the right to inspect, copy, and amend their PHI
  - Patients have a right to a list of all disclosures of their PHI
    - Exception: Some disclosures are permitted without the individual's authorization because they may have an effect on public health and safety
      - ❖ Reporting victims of abuse, neglect, or violence
      - ❖ Reporting of communicable and infectious disease
      - ❖ Court orders
      - ❖ Law enforcement purposes
      - ❖ Organ donation organizations
      - ❖ Medical examiners
      - ❖ Funeral directors
- Right to file a grievance or complaint with the practice or the organization's privacy officer
- Right to continuity of care
  - Continuous, cooperative provider/patient relationship
  - Exceptions:
    - Patient no longer requires treatment
    - Provider chooses to withdraw care due to noncompliant patient
      - ❖ Provider must notify the patient in writing that he is discontinuing care
      - ❖ Provider must refer patient to another physician
        - This protocol must be followed or the provider risks legal action for ending the provider/patient relationship without proper notice and a referral

---

11

WHAT:	**HIPAA PRIVACY RULE**
WHY:	**Protection of privacy**
	Safeguard information

HIPAA establishes national standards to protect individuals' medical records and other personal health information and applies to health plans, health care clearinghouses, and those health care providers who conduct certain health care transactions electronically. The Rule requires appropriate safeguards to protect the privacy of personal health information and sets limits and conditions on the uses and disclosures that may be made of such information without patient authorization. (http.//www.hhs.gov)

- Provides patients with certain rights known as Patient Privacy Rights that are communicated to the patient via the Notice of Privacy Practices
- Ensures reasonable and appropriate safeguards are implemented to protect the security and integrity of PHI

WHAT:	**JOINT COMMISSION**
WHY:	**Quality**
	Accreditation
	Reimbursement

An independent, not-for-profit organization, the Joint Commission (JC) accredits and certifies more than 19,000 health care organizations in the United States. Joint Commission accreditation is recognized nationwide as a symbol of quality that reflects an organization's commitment to meeting certain performance standards. Joint Commission standards are the basis of an objective evaluation process that can help health care organizations measure, access and improve performance. (http.//www.jointcommission.org)

- Formerly known as JCAHO (Joint Commission on the Accreditation of Health Care Organizations)
- Goal is to elevate the standards of health-care delivery
- Joint Commission accreditation is:
    - A condition of licensure in many states
    - A requirement for reimbursement by most third-party payers
    - Enhances staff recruitment by attracting highly qualified candidates

WHAT:	**EMTALA**
WHY:	**Human compassion**
	Treatment
	Liability

EMTALA (Emergency Medical Treatment and Active Labor Act) states that any patient who "comes to the emergency department" requesting "examination and treatment" must be provided with "an appropriate screening examination" to determine if he is suffering from an "emergency medical condition." If the patient is found to be experiencing an emergency medical condition, the hospital is obligated to provide him treatment until he is stable. If the hospital is unable to stabilize the patient, an appropriate transfer should be implemented. (http.//www.cms.gov)

- Passed as part of the Consolidated Omnibus Budget and Reconciliation Act of 1986 and sometimes referred to as the "Cobra Law," or the "Patient Anti-Dumping Law."
- States that no one who comes to the emergency department can be denied medical treatment based on citizenship, race, religion, or the ability to pay

WHAT:	**OSHA**
WHY:	**Safety**
	Education
	Training

OSHA (Occupational Safety and Health Administration) was established to prevent work injury, disability, illness, and death by enforcing rules and setting standards for workforce safety. Under the OSHA Act, employers are responsible for providing a safe and healthful workplace. OSHA offers a wide selection of training courses and educational programs to help broaden worker and employer knowledge on the recognition, avoidance, and prevention of safety and health hazards. (http.//www.osha.gov)

- Federal agency of the Department of Labor
- Assists state governments in their efforts to promote and assure safe and healthful working conditions
- Employers must comply with all applicable OSHA rules and standards

MY KEY NOTES

Part III

Front Office Fundamentals

The medical office team is made up of two types of personnel:

Clinical staff:

- Employees involved in direct patient care, such as doctors, nurses, and medical assistants.
- Primary focus is on care and treatment: record vital signs, perform examinations, diagnose diseases and disorders, administer tests, dispense medications and provide patient education.

Administrative staff:

- Office members who are not involved in direct patient care, such as front desk personnel, medical records specialists, coders, billers, and office coordinators.
- Primary focus is clerical and administrative duties: appointment scheduling, patient registration, coding, claims submission, reimbursement, and compliance.

WHO'S WHO IN THE MEDICAL OFFICE
Clinical Staff

Medical Doctor (MD) & Doctor of Osteopathy (DO):
- Diagnoses and treats disease, illness, and injury
- Prescribes medication and orders tests
- Establishes of plan of care
- Education:
  - Four years undergraduate work
  - Four years medical school
  - Three to eight years internship and residency
- ❖ *Doctor of Osteopathy is a Medical Doctor who has completed additional training in the musculoskeletal system.*

Physician Assistant (PA):
- Practices medicine under the supervision of a licensed physician
- Prescribes medication
- Education
  - Four years undergraduate work
  - Two to three years physician assistant training

Advanced Practice Nurse (APN) / Nurse Practitioner (NP):
- Serves in the capacity of a healthcare provider
- Prescribes medication (most states)
- Education
  - Four years undergraduate work
  - Master's degree in nursing

Registered Nurse (RN):
- Administers medications, treatments, and tests
- Establishes or contributes to an existing plan of care
- Provides information, education, and support to patients and families
- Education
  - Two-year associate of nursing degree (ADN) *or*
  - Three-year diploma school (RN) *or*
  - Four-year bachelor of science degree (BSN)

Licensed Practical Nurse (LPN) / Licensed Vocational Nurse (LVN):

- Provides basic patient care under the supervision of a physician or registered nurse
- Administers injections and applies dressings
- Collects data such as patient health history
- Education
  - One-year study in hospital, vocational school, or community college

Medical Assistant (MA):

- Records patients' vital signs and chief complaint for visit
- Prepares patients for examination and treatment
- Administers injections
- Education:
  - Training course in vocational high school program, certificate program, vocational school, or community college

Laboratory Technician:

- Obtains and prepares specimens and samples for testing and analysis
- Maintains inventory levels and equipment
- Education
  - Completion of an accredited laboratory technician program

CERTIFICATION, REGISTRATION & LICENSURE	
Certification	Individual has met predetermined educational and testing standards as specified by a professional association
Registration	Being placed on an official registry after meeting educational and testing requirements
Licensure	Individual has proper academic and clinical training in a specific field and has passed competency exams approved by the national certification organization

❖ *Certification, registration, and licensing requirements vary from state to state.*

WHO'S WHO IN THE MEDICAL OFFICE
Administrative Staff

Office Manager:
- Supervises staff
- Implements policy and procedure
- Oversees office to make sure it runs cost effectively and efficiently
- Ensures compliance with health, safety, and legal requirements

Front Office Staff:
- Greets and registers patients
- Schedules appointments
- Handle phones, messages, mail, and medical records
- Verifies insurance eligibility

Coder:
- Extracts information from the medical record and assigns standardized codes to diagnosis and procedures
- Reviews documentation for compliance and payer payment standards

Biller:
- Prepares and submits claims
- Generates patient statements
- Manages collections and claims denials

Medical Records Specialist:
- Maintains and organizes medical records
- Handles medical record requests
- Ensures databases are secure and only accessible to authorized personnel

Transcriptionist:
- Provides administrative support by transcribing dictation
- Creates text documents from dictated recordings
- Forwards finished documents to issuer for review and signature

❖ *Employer or health care system mandates education, certification, and experience for administrative staff*

Age-Related Care:

• Obstetrics	Pregnancy to birth
• Pediatrics	Birth through teens
• Family Medicine	Infants through adulthood
• Internal Medicine	Eighteen years old and up
• Geriatric Medicine	Sixty-five years old and up

Ambulatory Care:

Outpatient services that do not require an overnight hospital stay:

- Clinic service
- Diagnostic testing
- Laboratory
- Mental health counseling
- Physical therapy
- Primary care physician visit
- Radiology
- Specialist visit
- Surgery center

Emergency Care:

Medical or surgical conditions that require immediate care:

- Emergency room
- Urgent care

Continuing Care:

Long-term care for the elderly and patients with chronic conditions:

- Assisted living facility
- Nursing home

Hospice Care:

Caring for patients in the final stages of life, prognosis six months or less:

- Assisted living
- Home of patient, family, or friend
- Hospital
- Nursing home

Palliative Care:

Caring for patient with long-term, chronic conditions by providing comfort and relief from pain:

- Assisted living
- Home of patient, family, or friend
- Hospital
- Nursing home

Preventative Care:

Care provided to prevent disease:

- Health screenings
- Immunizations
- Patient education

Primary Care:

Health maintenance, diagnosis, and treatment of illness and disease:

- Primary care physician visit
- Specialist visit

Respite Care:

Providing downtime for caregivers by placing patient temporarily in care of someone else

- Short-term nursing home stay
- Twenty-four-hour home health care aide

Restorative Care:

Follow-up and rehabilitative care:

- Occupational therapy
- Physical therapy
- Rehabilitation center

Secondary Care:

Acute Care:

- Hospital admission

Tertiary Care:

Highly Specialized Care:

- Critical Care
- Intensive Care
- Surgery

Specialist	Specialty	Area of concentration
Audiologist	Audiology	Ears, hearing
Cardiologist	Cardiology	Heart, blood vessels
Dermatologist	Dermatology	Skin, hair, nails
Endocrinologist	Endocrinology	Glands, hormones
Gastroenterologist	Gastroenterology	Stomach, intestines
Gynecologist	Gynecology	Female reproductive system
Hematologist	Hematology	Blood, blood-forming organs
Nephrologist	Nephrology	Kidneys
Neurologist	Neurology	Brain, spinal cord
Obstetrician	Obstetrics	Pregnancy, childbirth
Oncologist	Oncology	Cancer
Ophthalmologist	Ophthalmology	Eyes, vision
Orthopedist	Orthopedics	Bones, muscles
Otolaryngologist	Otolaryngology	Ears, nose, throat
Podiatrist	Podiatry	Foot, ankle
Psychiatrist	Psychiatry	Mental health
Pulmonologist	Pulmonology	Lungs
Rheumatologist	Rheumatology	Joints, inflammation
Urologist	Urology	Urinary system & Male reproductive system

APPOINTMENT SCHEDULING
Key Terms

Diagnosis

Identification of disease or disorder from the signs and symptoms

Encounter Form

Billing form, also known as the charge slip or super-bill, that includes:
- Patient demographic information
- Patient type and reason for visit
- Provider name and identifier
- Evaluation and management code
- Diagnosis and procedure code
- Provider and patient signatures

Patient Demographics
- Information to identify the patient:
    - Name, address and phone number
    - Date of birth
    - E-mail address
    - Insurance information
- Information tracked for the purposes of statistical analysis and research:
    - Gender
    - Race
    - Ethnicity

Procedure

Surgical operation, technique, or service

Progress Notes

Summary of patient health status taken at each visit including:
- Reason for visit
- Scope of examination
- Diagnosis
- Treatment plan
- Medication (administered, prescribed, or renewed)
- Counseling/patient education
- Follow-up plan

Prognosis

Prediction of outcome or recovery from disease or illness; opinion on the course of disease

Scheduling is the assignment of an appropriate time slot to a patient appointment. Time slots must be accurately assigned. Overbooking can create long patient wait times, while under booking can result in low patient volume and lost revenue. Efficient appointment scheduling is critical to a successful practice. It ensures smooth office flow, provides for quality care, and contributes to physician productivity, employee morale, and patient satisfaction.

Patient Types

NEW:	New patient	First visit
EST:	Established patient	Previously seen
CONSULT:	Consultation	Patient referred to a specialist

Appointment Types

CON:	Consultation
BP:	Blood pressure check
EPI:	Episodic, sick
EKG:	Electrocardiogram
FU:	Follow up
GYN:	Pelvic exam
INJ:	Injection
LAB:	Blood draw
MVA:	Motor vehicle accident
NEW:	New patient
NRS:	Nurse visit
OV:	Office visit
PHY:	Physical
WC:	Workers' compensation
WI:	Walk-in

Appointment Scheduling

✓	Obtain:	Patient demographic and insurance information
✓	Verify:	Provider participates with patient insurance
✓	Determine:	Patient type and appointment type
✓	Access:	Provider schedule
✓	Enter:	Patient into the appropriate time slot
✓	Confirm:	Patient name, date, time, name of provider, and appointment location

Office visits, follow-ups, and episodic appointments are generally scheduled for ten to fifteen-minute time slots. New patient appointments, physicals, and consultations are usually scheduled for longer blocks of time. Every provider has his or her specific scheduling preferences.

PROVIDER SCHEDULE / AM SESSION:

TIME	PROVIDER	PATIENT TYPE	NAME	DOB	APPT TYPE
9:00	3210	EST	Cruz, Rosalie	10/03/39	OV
9:15	3210	EST	Cruz, Angel	02/08/38	OV
9:30	3210	EST	Black, Henry	04/23/58	WI
9:45	3210	NEW	Wills, Carol	12/29/73	NEW
10:00	3210	NEW	Wills, Carol	12/29/73	NEW
10:15	3210	EST	Cohen, Michael	05/12/86	FU
10:30	3210	EST	Adams, Jason	08/17/77	FU
10:45	3210	EST	Paulsen, Erika	10/01/55	EPI
11:00	3210	EST	Lee, Jessica	01/19/80	OV
11:15	3210	EST	Pinto, Anthony	07/14/81	PHY
11:30	3210	EST	Pinto, Anthony	07/14/81	PHY
11:45	3210	EST	Ryan, Joseph	05/15/95	EPI
12:00	3210	LUNCH			
12:15	3210	LUNCH			
12:30	3210	LUNCH			
12:45	3210	LUNCH			

PATIENT REGISTRATION

The goal of patient registration is to capture accurate and up-to-date patient demographics and confirm insurance eligibility. Incomplete, incorrect, or outdated data will impede the reimbursement process. Staff members who have a fundamental understanding of the cause and effect of registration on the cycle of reimbursement can prevent most claims denials.

New Patient
- Greet and welcome patient
- Provide patient with a copy of Notice of Privacy Practices
- Copy/scan photo ID
  - Validating a patient's identity is vital in the event there are several patients with the same name by making sure that an incorrect chart is not pulled in error
  - Ensures patient is not participating in an identify theft scheme
- Copy/scan both sides of the insurance card(s)
- Obtain referral, if applicable
- Provide patient with paperwork for completion
  - Patient registration form
  - Consent form(s)
  - Health history sheet
- Verify patient forms are complete and signed
- Enter patient information into system
- Confirm insurance eligibility
- Obtain patient signature on encounter form
- Collect copayment, if applicable, and provide receipt

Established Patient
- Greet and welcome patient
- Verify and update demographic information
- Confirm insurance eligibility
- Obtain referral, if applicable
- Obtain patient signature on encounter form
- Collect copayment, if applicable, and provide receipt

REGISTRATION FORM:

PATIENT INFORMATION
Health Park Family Medicine Center

Last name	First	M	Date
Ryan	Joseph	P	01/05/13

Date of Birth	E-mail	Phone
05/15/95	ryan@server.com	(555) 555-5555

Address	City, State	Zip code
123 Main Street	Centerton, NY	11111

Occupation	Employer
Student	N/A

Insurance Company	ID Number
NY Health HMO	ZZZ-111-222-AAA

Subscriber	Group Number:
Thomas Ryan	95-00000

Subscriber DOB:	Employer:
12/04/71	City of Centerton

Guarantor:	Relationship:	Phone:
Thomas Ryan	Father	(555) 555-1111

Secondary Insurance:	ID Number:
NY Health PPO	ZZZZ-222-333-DDD

Subscriber:	Group:
Mary Ryan	35-00000

Subscriber DOB:	Employer:
04/23/72	NY Medical Center

Emergency contact:	Relationship:	Phone:
Mary Ryan	Mother	(555) 555-5555

I authorize that my insurance benefits be paid directly to my physician. I understand that I am responsible for any balance.

Patient Signature: Mary Ryan/Mother   **Date :** 1/5/13

ENCOUNTER FORM:

PATIENT ENCOUNTER
Health Park Family Medicine Center

Date 01/05/13	Resource: 3210 P. Regan, MD	Facility: Park	Appt. Type: EPI: Sore throat

Name Joseph P. Ryan	Account 234477	DOB 05/15/95

Address 123 Main Street Centerton, NY 11111

Phone (555) 555-5555	Email joepryan51595@server.com

Insurance NY Health	ID Number ZZZ-111-222-AAA

Copay 20.00	Group 95-00000

E & M NEW Pt.		E & M Established Pt.		Procedures	
Low		Low		ECG interpret	
Low/Moderate		**Low/Moderate**	X	ECG rhythm	
Moderate		Moderate		Nebulizer	
Moderate/High		Moderate/High		Spirometer	
High		High		**Strep rapid**	**X**
Consultation		Consultation		UA complete	

Diagnosis					
Anemia		Fever		Palpitations	
Asthma		Headache		Pharyngitis	X
BPH		Hematuria		Pneumonia	
Bronchitis		Hyperlipidemia		Polyuria	
Conjunctivitis		Hypertension		Psoriasis	
Cystitis		Hyperthyroidism		PVD	
COPD		Hypothyroidism		Rhinitis	
Diabetes I		IBS		Sinusitis	
Diabetes II		Influenza		URI	
DVT		Insomnia		Urticaria	
Dysphagia		Laryngitis		UTI	
Emphysema		Migraine		Other	

Patient signature: Mary Ryan/Mother

Provider signature: P. Regan, MD

Date: 1/5/13

Next Appointment: PRN

Instructions: Rx: Amoxicillin

MEDICAL CHARTS
Key Terms

Electronic Medical Record
Medical chart in electronic form

Hybrid Chart
Medical chart that exists in both paper and electronic form

Medical Chart
Record of patient demographic and health information in paper or electronic form

Paper Chart
Medical chart in paper form

Purpose of the Medical Chart
The medical chart is a confidential and legal document containing patient demographic information, health history, and detailed documentation of care and treatment. It is a vital tool in evaluating and coordinating patient care, and essential for accreditation and reimbursement.

- Serves as a legal record of medical care and must contain:
    - Accurate information to identify the patient
    - Documentation to support diagnosis and to substantiate and justify treatment
    - Complete and comprehensive records to promote continuity of care among providers
- Also known as the medical record or health record
- May appear in paper or electronic form
- Organized using a tabular format

Chart Organization
Charts are divided into sections by the use of TABS. TABS are the key to chart uniformity and ensure that documents are organized in a consistent manner. Most practices customize TABS to reflect the specific needs of their practice. Some utilize only a few general TABS, while others incorporate numerous, more specific TABS. Each TAB represents a heading where documents are filed and retrieved.

CHART TABS:

TABS	DOCUMENTS
Advance Directive	Living will, medical power of attorney
Cardiology	Reports and summaries from cardiac testing
Consent Forms	Permission for care, treatment, and chart access
Consultation	Correspondence to and from referring specialists
Correspondence	General correspondence: employer, school, misc.
Demographics	Patient registration sheet, copy of photo ID
Diagnostic Testing	Results and summaries from diagnostic testing
Health History	Comprehensive record of patient health history
Immunizations	Immunization records
Insurance	Insurance coverage and benefit information
Laboratory	Reports from laboratory testing
Medications	Medications administered and prescribed
Pathology	Reports and summaries from pathology testing
Physical Exam	Notes from physical examinations
Progress Notes	Documentation taken at each visit
Radiology	Reports from x-ray and diagnostic testing
Referrals	Referrals issued and received

ELECTRONIC MEDICAL RECORDS (EMR)

Until recently, medical records were maintained in paper form, but due to advances in technology and pressure by government officials, they are transitioning to the Electronic Medical Record, a computer-based program.

	EMR	PAPER CHARTS
Location	The EMR is a complete and comprehensive record of patient information located in a central database.	Patient information in paper charts is often fragmented. Records are often spread among many providers and facilities.
Efficiency	The medical record is never lost or misfiled. Immediate access to information improves efficiency.	Patient charts are often misfiled or misplaced. Valuable time is spent trying to locate a missing record.
Access	The patient chart is available from any workstation. Multiple users can view the record at the same time.	Paper charts can only physically be in one place at a time. Requests for records by another provider must be copied or faxed.
Clarity	Information contained in the EMR is clear and legible.	Hand written entries are sometimes hard to decipher. This can contribute to medical errors.
Privacy	Access to patient records can be restricted and monitored. Unauthorized access can be tracked.	Paper charts do not contain any tracking method for unauthorized access.
Updates	As soon as patient information is entered into the EMR, it is available to all users.	Patient information must be updated with each individual provider to stay current.

DOCUMENTATION

Documentation is the written or electronically generated information about patient care. It is the basis for communication between physicians and other healthcare professionals.

Every member of the health care team should have a thorough understanding of chart documentation in order to maintain a clear and concise record. Although documentation is left to the clinical staff, it is necessary for front office personnel to know the format, terminology, abbreviations, and acronyms.

Purpose of Documentation

- Ensure accreditation
- Facilitate communication
- Satisfy compliance criterions
- Promote continuity of care
- Assist with education and research
- Requirement for reimbursement
- Meet professional and legal standards

Documentation Guidelines

- Documentation must be accurate, timely, correct, and complete
- Verify you have the correct patient chart by checking the name, date of birth, or patient identifiers
- Use only black ink
- Write legibly
- Include patient name or identifier on each page
- Include date on all records
- Predating or backdating an entry is unethical and illegal
- Document using chronological order
- Sign each entry; never use initials where a signature is required by law or regulation
- Never erase an entry
- Never use correction fluid on an entry
- If you make a mistake, cross it out in a single line and date and sign the correction
- Never leave blank spaces
- Avoid grammatical and spelling errors

Documentation Formats

SOAP Documentation:

S	**Subjective**	Symptoms:	What the patient tells you
O	**Objective**	Facts:	Test results
A	**Assessment**	Diagnosis:	Conclusion
P	**Plan**	Treatment:	Plan of care

PIE Documentation:

P	**Problem**	Identification of the problem
I	**Intervention**	Documentation of action taken
E	**Evaluation**	Determination of the success of the action

Documentation Abbreviations

BP	Blood Pressure
DDx	Differential Diagnosis
Dx	Diagnosis
FHx	Family History
H&P	History & Physical
HPI	History of Present Illness
MDM	Medical Decision Making
NKA	No Known Allergies
NKDA	No Known Drug Allergies
nl	Normal Limits
P	Pulse
PFSHx	Past Family & Social History
PMHx	Past Medical History
R/O	Rule Out
ROS	Review of Symptoms
S/S	Signs & Symptoms
Sx	Symptoms
Tx	Treatment
wnl	Within Normal Limits

MEDICAL TERMINOLOGY

Medical terminology is the language of medicine. It standardizes words and phrases to describe diseases, diagnoses, and procedures. Medical terms are built by combining word parts: prefixes, root words, and suffixes.

Prefixes
- Placed at the beginning of the word
- Usually refers to number, location, or time
- Not every medical term has a prefix

ab:	away from	macro:	large
ante:	before	mal:	bad
anti:	against	micro:	small
brady:	slow	para:	around
dia:	through	pluri:	several
dys:	abnormal	poly:	many
end:	within	post:	after
epi:	above, upon	pre:	before
exo:	out of, away	pro:	in front of
hyper:	high	sub:	under
hypo:	low	tachy:	fast

Root Words
- Base of the word
- Usually describes a part of the body or the body system
- Some medical terms have more than one root word

abdomin/o:	abdomen	glyc/o:	sugar
aden/o:	gland	hemat/o:	blood
audi/o:	ear	hepat/o:	liver
cardi/o:	heart	lipid/o:	fat
cervic/o:	neck	my/o:	muscle
col/o:	colon	nephr/o:	kidney
cyst/o:	bladder	ocul/o:	eye
dermat/o:	skin	neur/o:	nerve
encephala/o:	brain	oste/o:	bone
enter/o:	intestine	pulmon/o:	lung
gastr/o:	stomach	ven/o:	vein

Linking Vowels
- Linking vowels link the root word to another root word or suffix
- The most common vowel used is o

Suffixes
- Placed at the end of the root word
- Usually refers to disease, condition, or procedure
- Every medical term has a suffix

algia:	pain	itis:	inflamed
cele:	swelling	logy:	study of
centesis:	puncture	pathy:	disease
ectomy:	removal	penia:	decrease
edema:	swelling	pepsia:	digestion
emia:	blood	pexy:	fixation
gram:	picture	phagia:	swallow
graphy:	recording	scopy:	view
ia:	condition	stenosis:	narrow
ist:	specialist	therapy:	treatment

TERM	PREFIX	ROOT	SUFFIX	MEANING
gastritis		gastr/o	itis	inflammation of the stomach
bradycardia	brady	cardi/o	ia	fast heartbeat
tachycardia	tachy	cardi/o	ia	slow heartbeat
hyperglycemia	hyper	glyc/o	emia	high blood sugar condition
hypoglycemia	hypo	glyc/o	emia	low blood sugar condition
hyperlipidemia	hyper	lip/o	emia	high fat levels in blood
hypolipidemia	hypo	lip/o	emia	low fat levels in blood
myalgia		my/o	algia	muscle pain
cardiomyopathy		cardi/o my/o	pathy	disease of the heart muscle

MEDICAL RECORDS
Key Terms

Active Chart
Chart of a patient currently receiving care

Authorization Form
Customized document giving permission for a specific purpose

Closed Chart
Chart of a patient who has died, transferred, or moved away

Complete Chart
Chart that contains complete and accurate documentation

Delinquent Chart
Chart that remains incomplete longer than the guidelines established by laws and regulations

Inactive Chart
Chart of a patient who has not been seen in a year or more

Incomplete Chart
Chart containing deficiencies in documentation and missing information

Protocol
Established guidelines

Medical Record Contents
The medical record is a permanent and legal documentation of medical treatment, and should contain accurate information to identify the patient, support the diagnosis, and document a plan of care:

- Advance directive
- Consent forms
- Health history
- Insurance information
- Patient demographics
- Progress notes
- Referrals
- Tests results

The protected health information it contains is confidential and protected by law from unauthorized disclosure. Employees are obligated to safeguard and protect the medical record. It is their legal and ethical responsibility to treat records with complete confidentiality.

Ownership
The medical chart is the property of the provider that created the record. Providers are required by law to create, maintain and retain them. Under HIPAA, patients have the right to access and copy their protected health information.

PHI in the Medical Office

- Use PHI only when it is necessary to perform your job duties
- Only access information that is relevant to patient care
- Do not discuss PHI with anyone unless it is required of your job
- Always be aware of where you are and who is around when discussing PHI
- Try to choose a private area and never discuss PHI in public places
- Lower your voice when discussing PHI on the telephone
- Do not leave PHI where patients or visitors can see it
- Ensure computer screens are not visible to passersby, or install a privacy screen
- Use cover sheets with a **CONFIDENTIAL** heading on outgoing faxes transmitting PHI
- Check printers, copiers, and fax machines for documents when you are finished using them
- Never throw away PHI; always shred or place in a secure bin

Medical Record Maintenance and Retention

- Records must be kept for every patient treated
- Maintained in their entirety; no documents should be permanently removed or deleted
- Stored in a safe and secure area that provides protection from loss, damage, and unauthorized access
- Retained in accordance with state and federal regulations:
  - To secure continuity of patient care
  - For research and education purposes
  - To record outcomes of treatment

Authorization to Release Information Form

- Must be informed consent and include:
  - Name of provider or practice releasing the information
  - Name of the provider, facility, or agency receiving information
  - Patient name, address, and date of birth
  - Purpose of the information
  - How much information is to be released
  - Effective and expiration dates of the consent
  - Signature of patient or legal representative

AUTHORIZATION TO RELEASE PHI FORM:

Authorization to Release
PROTECTED HEALTH INFORMATION
Health Park Family Medicine

Patient Name: _____ Date of Birth: _____

Address: _____ Telephone: _____

I, _____

authorize, _____

to release my health care information to:

Name: _____

Address: _____

City, State, Zip Code: _____

Telephone: _____

This request applies to:

□ Complete medical record

□ Health care information limited to the following condition or dates:

_____

Reason /Purpose for Disclosure:
□ Medical

□ Legal

□ Financial

□ Personal

I have read and understood the information in this authorization.

Patient Signature _____ Date _____

This authorization expires one year from today

REIMBURSEMENT
Key Terms

Charge Entry
Entering patient charges for services rendered into a database ·

Claim
Form submitted to a third party payer by a healthcare provider or patient requesting payment or reimbursement

Clean Claim
Claim that is complete and correct

Reimbursement
Receiving payment for services rendered

Rejected Claim
Claim denied reimbursement due to incompleteness or error

Reimbursement Process
- Patient demographic and insurance information are verified
- Service is provided to patient
- Encounter is completed and coded correctly
- Claim is submitted appropriately
- Health plan issues payment

Staff Roles in Reimbursement
- Front Office Staff:
  - Enters and verifies patient account information
  - Confirms insurance coverage and eligibility
- Provider:
  - Documents elements of patient visit in progress notes
  - Completes encounter form accurately and completely
- Coder & Biller:
  - Confirms provider documentation supports the services
  - Extracts and assigns codes
- Biller:
  - Submits claims and generates statements
  - Reviews payments and manages claims denials

Claims submissions to insurance companies must be timely, complete, and correct. Errors and omissions are costly and expensive. Without accurate patient demographics, insurance information, and proper coding, the insurance company will not pay the claim, or will pay less than the provider is entitled to receive. When a claim is incomplete, it will fail and must be resubmitted. This requires additional time and delays payment.

Alphabetical

Alphabetize the names of individuals by last name, first name, and then middle:

- Reynolds, Anne M.
- Reynolds, Anne Marie
- Reynolds, Anne Mary

Treat hyphenated or compound words as one word:

- Smith Jones, David F.
- Smith-Jones, David N.
- Smith Jones, Donna K.

Alphabetize abbreviated prefixes such as St. according the complete spelling of the word Saint:

- Saint John, Paul
- St. John, Paula
- Saint John, Phillip

Ignore capitalization in surnames having prefixes such as Mac and Mc, and file just as they are spelled:

- MacDonald, William
- MacDougall, Patricia
- McDougall, Patrick

Numerical

Straight numerical: assignment of sequential numbers:

- 123456
- 123457
- 123458
- 123459
- 123460
- 123461

Digit Methods: numbers are divided into three groups of two digit numbers:

- 12-34-56
- 12-34-57
- 12-34-58
- 12-34-59
- 12-34-60
- 12-34-61

TELEPHONES

The front office staff is the first point of contact an individual has with the medical office. They are responsible for providing a good first impression and projecting a positive and professional image.

- Before sitting down to answer the phones for the first time, familiarize yourself with how the phone system works. This will prevent calls from being disconnected or transferred incorrectly. Know:
  - Standard practice greeting for answering the phone
  - How to put a call on hold
  - How to transfer a call
  - How, and at what times, to put phones on and take phones off service
  - Name, number, and procedure for accessing the answering service and messages
  - How to handle emergency calls according to office protocol:
    - *What to do if a patient is complaining of chest pain*
    - *What to do if a lab is calling with critical lab results on a patient*
- Place a mirror near the telephone to see how you look when you answer; make every effort to have a smile in your voice each time you pick up the phone
- Answer the phone as promptly as possible
- Make sure to identify yourself and the name of your practice or organization
- Always be pleasant and considerate; incorporate words like please, thank you, hello, goodbye, certainly, glad, understandable, and my pleasure
- Do not rush the caller; take the time to make him feel valued and respected
- Listen to the caller and focus on why he is calling in order to assist or direct him to the proper person
- Always ask before putting someone on hold; when you pick the line up again, thank him for holding
- Ask the caller's name before transferring a call and announce the caller by name to whom you are transferring the call before completing the transfer
- Have the necessary information, directories, and resources at hand to be able to articulately answer frequently asked questions

Messages should be clear, concise, and easy to decipher:

- Write legibly
- Color code messages if there is more than one provider
- Record the date and time
- Obtain the full name of the caller and verify the spelling
- Obtain the company name if applicable
- Obtain and confirm the call back number
- Read the message back to the caller to make sure the details are complete and accurate
- Record what action needs to be taken for the recipient of the message:
  - Urgent
  - Caller will call back in the morning
  - Please return call
- Tell the caller the action you will take:
  - I will leave the message on his desk
  - I will give him the message when he is back in the office on Monday
- Avoid using scraps of paper to record messages; they are easily misplaced and sometimes hard to read
- Always sign or initial the message in the event the recipient needs clarification or additional information
- Leave the message in a designated area for the recipient
- Deliver messages in a timely manner

TO:	Dr. Regan	DATE:	01/05/13
FROM:	Erika Paulsen	TIME:	9:45 AM
Phone:	555-5555	RECORDED BY:	Ashley B

Samples of allergy med. Clarity 20 mg. provided at recent appt. are working. Patient req. RX for 90-day supply phoned into Centerton Pharmacy
Patient DOB: 10/1/55   Pharmacy: # 555-4444

MY KEY NOTES

Part IV
Medical Coding 101

Who:

Medical and Health Organizations including:

- American Medical Association (AMA)
- Centers for Medicare and Medicaid Services (CMS)
- World Health Organization (WHO)

What:

Developed and implemented medical coding classification systems:

- ICD-9 CM: International Classification of Diseases Ninth Revision, Clinical Modification
  - Codes diagnosis
- CPT-4: Current Procedural Terminology Fourth Edition
  - Codes procedures
- HCPCS: Healthcare Common Procedure Coding System
  - Codes hospital outpatient and physician services

Why:

To create a uniform and universally recognized medical language

How:

By translating written information of diseases, symptoms, injuries, illnesses, and services into numeric codes

MEDICAL CODING

Medical coding is the process of assigning standardized numeric codes to diagnoses, procedures, and services. Doing so creates a single language by which all providers, insurance companies, and government agencies can communicate.

- Ensures uniform communication among providers
- Allows for monitoring the quality of patient care
- Fundamental requirement for reimbursement
- Standardizes billing by establishing consistent reimbursement fees
- Facilitates universal reporting of morbidity (illness and disease) and mortality (death) rates
- Provides statistical information for quality control and management purposes
- Supports funding and research
- Evaluates processes and outcomes in health care
- Helps predict trends in health care and plan for future health care needs

ICD-9 CM CODES

ICD-9 CM is the International Classification of Diseases Ninth Revision, Clinical Modification:
- Used to code:
  - Condition
  - Diagnosis
  - Disease
  - Injury
  - Signs
  - Symptoms
- Describes *why*
- Three to five-digit codes
- Divided into three volumes:
  - Volume 1: Tabular Index of Disease
  - Volume 2: Alphabetical Index of Disease
  - Volume 3: Tabular and Alphabetical Indexes for Procedure Classification (codes inpatient hospital stays)

VOLUME 1: TABULAR INDEX OF DISEASE:

CODE RANGE	DIAGNOSIS
001–139	Infectious and parasitic diseases
140–239	Neoplasms
240–279	Endocrine, nutritional, metabolic diseases, and immunity disorders
280–289	Diseases of the blood-forming organs
290–319	Mental disorders
320–359	Diseases of the nervous system
360–389	Diseases of the sense organs
390–459	Diseases of the circulatory system
460–519	Diseases of the respiratory system
520–579	Diseases of the digestive system
580–629	Diseases of the genitourinary system
630–679	Complications of pregnancy, childbirth, and puerperium
680–709	Diseases of the skin and subcutaneous tissue
710–739	Diseases of the musculoskeletal system and connective tissue
740–759	Congenital anomalies
760–779	Certain conditions originating in the perinatal period
780–799	Symptoms, signs, and ill-defined conditions
800–899	Injury and poisoning

Diagnosis Guidelines
- Primary diagnosis   Chief complaint (CC) or main reason
- Secondary diagnosis   Additional complaint or coexisting reason
- Tertiary Diagnosis   Third reason

Coding to the highest degree of specialization
ICD-9 CM codes range from three to five digits. Coding out to five digits is referred to as coding to the highest degree of specialization. Code to the highest degree whenever possible.
- Three-digit codes are *General* codes
- Four-digit codes are *Specific* codes
- Five-digit codes are *Most Specific* codes

DIAGNOSIS	CODE	SPECIFICITY
Anemia	285	General Three-digit code
Anemia in chronic disease	285.2	Specific Four-digit code
Anemia in chronic kidney disease	285.21	Most specific Five-digit code

V Codes: Health status and contact with health services codes
- V codes are used to describe an encounter between a provider and an *individual without an active illness*.
- They are used for someone who is not sick, but who is receiving medical care:
  - Counseling
  - Health screenings
  - Prenatal check ups and well-baby visits
  - Preventative medicine
  - Suture removal
  - Vaccinations

E Codes: External causes of injury and poisoning codes

- E codes explain *how and where* the initial encounter of an injury or poisoning happened:
  - Accidental drowning
  - Accidents due to natural and environmental factors
  - Airplane accidents
  - Injuries from a fall
  - Injuries from fire
  - Motor vehicle accidents
  - Railway accidents
  - Water transport accidents
- E codes help the coder identify the correct insurance carrier for the claim
- E codes are *only* used by the initial provider or entity that saw the patient
- E codes are *never* used as a primary diagnosis, but they may be used as a supplemental or additional diagnosis

ICD-10-CM Implementation

The United States Department of Health and Human Services will be replacing the ICD-9-CM code set with the ICD-10-CM code set in 2014. ICD-10-CM was developed by the Centers for Disease Control and Prevention for use in all healthcare settings. As a result of new technology and scientific advancements in medicine, the new ICD-10 classification system will be expanded to reflect greater specificity and more detailed information. Terminology and disease classifications have been updated to reflect current and emerging conditions and needs.

- Number of available codes will increase from approximately 13,000 to about 69,000
- Code book chapters will expand from 17 to about 21
- Diagnosis codes will change from the current numeric three to five-digit codes to alpha-numeric three to seven-digit codes
- Longer code descriptions will provide for greater clinical detail and specificity and reduce the need to include supporting documentation with claims
- The new format will allow for the easy incorporation of new codes and assist with public health reporting and tracking

CPT-4 is the Current Procedural Terminology Fourth Edition

- Used to code medical, surgical, and diagnostic procedures
- Describes *what*
- Five-digit codes

CODE RANGE	PROCEDURE TYPE
00100–01999, 99100–99150	Anesthesia Codes
10021–69990	Surgery Codes
70010–79999	Radiology Codes
80047–89398, 99500–99607	Medicine Codes
99201–99499	Evaluation and Management Codes

Evaluation and Management (E&M) codes include:

- Outpatient services
- Hospital or inpatient services
- Preventative medical services
- Provider office visits

E&M provider office visit codes are determined by several components:

- Complexity of medical decision-making
- Counseling
- Examination
- History of present illness
- Patient education
- Patient health history
- Review of symptoms
- Time spent "face-to-face" with patient

Collectively these components are known as Level Of Care (LOC):

LEVEL OF CARE	NEW PATIENT E&M CODES	ESTABLISHED PATIENT E&M CODES
LOW Ten Minutes	99201	99211
LOW/MODERATE Twenty Minutes	99202	99212
MODERATE Thirty Minutes	99203	99213
MODERATE/HIGH Forty-five Minutes	99204	99214
HIGH Sixty Minutes	99205	99215

The Centers for Medicare and Medicaid Services (CMS) have developed specific guidelines and documentation requirements for evaluation and management codes. There are different codes for each procedure. Providers must select the one that best represents the time and services provided during the patient visit.

J Codes: Drug injections and administration codes include:

- Acetaminophen injection
- Epinephrine injection
- Inhalation solution
- Lidocaine injection
- Penicillin injection

G Codes: Medicare preventative services codes include:

- Welcome to Medicare exam
- Annual wellness visit
- Pap smear
- Pelvic and breast exam
- Prostate/PSA exam

CODING GUIDELINES

Always code from a current edition of the ICD-9 CM and CPT-4; coding books are updated annually and revised periodically.

- Codes must accurately reflect only the services that were provided
- Codes must be supported by documentation
- Always code to the highest degree of specialization to ensure proper reimbursement; fourth and fifth digit sub-classification codes must be used whenever possible
- The responsibility of accurately capturing diagnoses and procedures lies with the provider, not the coder; query the provider if you need clarification or additional information

Assigning diagnosis codes

1. Find: Diagnosis on the encounter form or in the progress notes
2. Locate: Diagnosis in the alphabetical index of the ICD-9 CM and choose a tentative code
3. Utilize: Cross reference instructions if the code is not found under the first entry
4. Reference: Tabular index of the ICD-9 CM to verify that this is still the most accurate code
5. Assign: Select and assign the most appropriate code

Modifiers

Modifiers are two-digit codes that are sometimes used in conjunction with CPT-4 codes. They indicate that a service was altered in some way from the stated code descriptor by providing supplemental information to insurance companies. They provide justification as to why the additional procedures should be paid.

- Explain certain circumstances or conditions of patient care
- Allow the provider to bill for multiple procedures on the same day of service
- Signify that only part of a service was performed
- Specify a service or procedure was increased or decreased
- Indicate a repeat or multiple procedure
- Determine reimbursement rates; correct use of modifiers increase reimbursement, while improper use can result in loss of revenue, overpayment, or denial of a claim

CODING COMPLIANCE

Third-party payers dictate that providers adhere to specific coding guidelines to guarantee payment. Coding compliance is a system of internal checks and balances that ensure rules and regulations are followed.

Medical Necessity Rule

The Medical Necessity Rule states that medical services provided must be supported by an appropriate diagnosis to ensure reimbursement by third-party payers.

Scenario 1:

- A provider orders an EKG (heart test) on a patient complaining of knee pain, and the patient has no risk factors presenting for heart disease
- EKG (service) does not support knee pain (diagnosis)
- Insurance company will not pay the cost of the EKG because the diagnosis does not support the procedure; therefore, it is not considered a medical necessity

Scenario 2:

- A provider orders an EKG on a patient complaining of heart palpitations (warning sign of a heart condition)
- EKG (service) supports heart palpitations (diagnosis)
- Insurance company will pay the cost of the EKG because it supported the diagnosis; therefore, it is considered a medical necessity

Illegal billing practices

Coding for Coverage	Using a code that is not the most accurate, but one that the insurance company will reimburse for; misrepresenting a code to justify treatment
Up Coding	Using a higher E&M code, rather than the most appropriate, with the intention of increasing reimbursement
Unbundling	Dividing and submitting services into separate codes when only a single CPT-4 code is necessary

MY KEY NOTES

Part V

Introduction to Health Insurance

Health insurance falls into two categories:

Private/Commercial Health Insurance

- Managed Care Organizations
- Fee for Service
- Health Savings and Spending Accounts

Public/Government Programs

- Children's Health Insurance Program
- Federal Employees Health Benefits Program
- Indian Health Service
- Medicaid
- Medicare
- Military Insurance

HEALTH INSURANCE
Key Terms

Advance Beneficiary Notice (ABN)
Notice given to Medicare patients that insurance may not cover a certain service. By signing the form, the patient agrees to be financially responsible if Medicare denies payment.

Capitation
Fixed, prepaid premium

COBRA
Consolidated Omnibus Reconciliation Act. Health insurance coverage available to individuals and their dependents when they leave their place of employment; prevents a lapse in health insurance coverage

Coinsurance
Percentage or the amount of the bill the patient is responsible for

Copay
Amount paid by patient at each provider visit as mandated by their insurance plan

Deductible
Amount a patient must pay for medical services before their health plan will cover any costs

Pre-Authorization
Approval by an insurance company for a provider to render a specific health care service to the patient

Pre-Certification
Procedure for reviewing the appropriateness and medical necessity of a healthcare service

Referral
Authorization issued by a primary care physician that allows the patient to receive additional care through a specialist

Second Surgical Opinion
Encourages or requires a patient to obtain the opinion of another provider after their physician has recommended a non-emergency surgery or outpatient elective surgery

Utilization Review
Review of patient healthcare services to make sure they agree with the standards set by the managed care organization; a tracking method used to record the medical necessity of a service

Affiliated Provider	Health care provider contracted with a Managed Care Organization (MCO)
Beneficiary	Individual who is covered and receives benefits through an insurance policy; any eligible person, subscriber, enrollee, member, or dependent
Carrier	The insurance company or government agency that finances and administers the health insurance plan
Claimant	Person or entity submitting a claim
Decedent	Deceased individual
Dependent	Spouse and/or unmarried children (natural, adopted, or step) of an insured
Enrollee	Member receiving services under a health plan; an eligible person who is enrolled in a health insurance plan
Gatekeeper	Term used to describe the Primary Care Provider (PCP) in a Health Management Organization (HMO); role is to coordinate health care for members
Guarantor	Person who guarantees to pay the provider whatever the insurance company does not pay; also known as the responsible party
Insured	Person covered by a health insurance policy
Insurer	Insurance company or government agency providing the health plan
Member	Anyone covered under a health insurance plan
Network Provider	Provider contracted with a Managed Care Organization to provide service to its members
Non-participating Provider	Provider who has not contracted with a Managed Care Organization

Patient	Person receiving health care benefits
Plan Administrator	Individual, firm or company designated by your health plan or employer to handle record keeping and claims submission
Plan Participant	Employee, beneficiary, or dependent of the employee receiving benefits
Preferred Provider	Provider who has contracted with a MCO and participates on most levels
Primary Care Provider	Provider who coordinates a patient's primary care; also known as the primary care physician
Provider	Broad term used for health professionals who provide health care services; the term refers to physicians, hospitals, and ancillary services
Provider Network	Healthcare providers contracted with a Managed Care Organization to provide service to its members
Responsible Party	Person who agrees to pay the provider whatever the insurance company does not pay; also known as the guarantor
Specialist	Doctor trained in a specific type of medicine
Subscriber	Person or organization that pays for the insurance; person whose employment makes him or her eligible for group insurance
Third Party Administrator	An individual, firm or insurance company hired by the employer to handle claims and pay providers
Third Party Payer	Entity other than the patient (first party) and the provider (second party) involved with health care financing
Underinsured	Individual with private or government insurance that does not cover all patient health care costs
Uninsured	Person who is not covered by any health insurance policy

PRIVATE & COMMERCIAL
HEALTH INSURANCE

I. MANAGED CARE

Health insurance plans that are contracted with providers (physicians, hospitals, labs) to provide care for members at a reduced rate. The contracted providers make up the plans network. Types of managed care organizations include:

- Health Maintenance Organization (HMO)
- Preferred Provider Organization (PPO)
- Point of Service (POS)
- Exclusive Provider Organization (EPO)

Health Maintenance Organization Models

Staff	Physicians are salaried and work as direct employees of the health maintenance organization
Group	Health maintenance organization does not pay the physician directly but, instead, pays the physician group
Open-Panel	Physician maintains his or her own office but also sees non-HMO patients
Network	Health maintenance organization contracts with both physician groups and individual practices

Health Maintenance Organization (HMO)
Overview

- HMOs provide medical services on a prepaid basis
- Patients must use network providers
- Requires seeing your primary care physician (PCP) before a referral is issued to a specialist

In Network

- Requires choosing a PCP/gatekeeper
- Copayment is due at time of service
- Little or no paperwork
- Required to see only providers contracted by the health maintenance organization

Out of Network

- Must pay out of pocket
- No reimbursement for out of network providers except for emergencies outside the HMO area

Preferred Provider Organization (PPO)

Overview

- Network providers charge on a fee-for-service basis but are paid on a discounted fee schedule

In Network

- Patients do not need to choose a PCP, but the physician must be in network
- Referrals to specialists are not required

Out of Network

- If you go out of network, you must pay out of pocket and then submit the bill to the insurance company and wait for reimbursement; you will be paid at a reduced rate
- Expenses for emergency care outside of area are reimbursed

Point Of Service (POS)

Overview

- POS is a hybrid between an HMO plan and a Fee for Service (indemnity) plan that allows members to seek treatment from a non-participating provider but at a lower level of benefits

In Network

- Must choose a PCP/gatekeeper
- Must obtain a referral from PCP before seeing a specialist
- Little or no paperwork

Out of Network

- Can see any provider you like
- No referral is required
- Substantially higher out-of-pocket costs
- Must submit claim forms and bills to insurance company

Exclusive Provider Organization (EPO)

Overview

- Network or group of providers who have contracted with an insurance company to provide health care services to subscribers at significantly lower rates

In Network

- Must use network providers
- Must choose a PCP/gatekeeper
- Must obtain a referral before seeing a specialist

Out of Network

- No reimbursement, except for emergency care outside the area
- High out-of-pocket costs

II. HEALTH SAVING AND SPENDING ACCOUNTS

Plans designed to help individuals pay for healthcare. They work in combination with a high deductible health insurance plan. The primary purpose is to pay for qualified medical expenses tax-free. Types of savings and spending plans include:

- Health Savings Accounts (HSA)
- Medical Savings Accounts (MSA)
- Flexible Spending Accounts (FSA)

Health Savings Account (HSA)

- Tax-exempt trust or custodial account that you set up with a qualified health saving account trustee to pay or reimburse certain medical expenses
- Individuals covered by high-deductible health plans receive tax-deferred treatment of money saved for medical expenses

Medical Savings Account (MSA)

- MSAs are medical plans that combine high-deductible insurance protection with a tax-deferred savings account
- Participants pay healthcare expenses from this account up to the amount of the insurance deductible

Flexible Spending Account (FSA)

- Employees are reimbursed for medical expenses
- Usually funded through voluntary salary deduction agreements with employer who may also contribute
- No employment or federal taxes are deducted from your contribution

III. FEE FOR SERVICE

Fee for Service plans offer flexibility of choice in exchange for higher out-of-pocket expenses and more paperwork. Members pay for services up front and then submit a claim form to the insurance company for reimbursement. Medical costs are split between the insurance plan and the subscriber, with each paying a fixed percentage. Individuals can choose their own providers. There are no networks. Most plans have a deductible. They are also known as:

- Indemnity insurance
- Major medical insurance
- Traditional insurance

PUBLIC & GOVERNMENT
HEALTH INSURANCE

I. MEDICARE
Federal program administered by the Centers for Medicare and Medicaid Services that provides care to individuals without regard to income or medical history.
- Helps pay for a range of medical services, including hospital, physician, home health care, diagnostic tests and prescription drugs for:
  - Individuals sixty-five or older
  - Individuals with long-term disabilities
  - Individuals with End-Stage Renal Disease (ESRD)

Part A: Hospital Coverage
- Hospital stay
- Skilled nursing home care following a hospital stay
- Home health care following a hospital stay
- Hospice care

Part B: Medical Outpatient Insurance
- Diagnostic testing
- Durable medical equipment
- Laboratory testing
- Mental health services
- Outpatient surgery
- Physical therapy
- Preventative services
- Provider office visits
- Specialist office visits

Part C: Medicare Advantage Plan
- Includes both Part A (Hospital Insurance) and Part B (Outpatient Insurance)
- Most people pay a monthly premium, the Part B premium, and a copayment (if required by their specific plan) for covered services

Part D: Prescription Drug Coverage
- Medicare Advantage Plans usually include a drug plan for an additional cost
- Original Medicare offers drug plans through Medicare-approved insurance companies or private companies at an added cost

MEDIGAP: Medicare Supplemental Insurance

- Optional private insurance that fills in the gap on original Medicare coverage
- Individual must have Part A and Part B to buy a Medigap policy
- Medigap pays copayments and deductibles

Services are not covered by Medicare A & B

- Acupuncture
- Chiropractic services
- Cosmetic surgery
- Deductibles, coinsurance, or copayments
- Dental care
- Eye care
- Hearing aids
- Long-term care
- Prescription drugs
- Routine foot care

II. MEDICAID

Program based on federal guidelines and administered at the state level. Each state oversees its own eligibility standards and program.

- Provides health care coverage to low-income individuals, families, the aged, blind and disabled
- Coverage includes:
  - Ambulatory care
  - Clinic services
  - Diagnostic testing
  - Family planning services
  - Home health services
  - Hospital care
  - Laboratory testing
  - Medical equipment
  - Nursing home care
  - Prenatal care
  - Preventative care
  - Vaccinations

III. CHILDREN'S HEALTH INSURANCE PROGRAM (CHIP)

- Federal government program administered at the state level
- Provides health care for low-income children whose parents do not qualify for Medicaid but who cannot afford private insurance

IV. INDIAN HEALTH SERVICE (IHS)

- Program administered through the Department of Health and Human Services
- Provides medical care to eligible American Indians and Alaskan natives

V. FEDERAL EMPLOYEES HEALTH BENEFITS (FEHB)

- Program administered by the United States Office of Personnel Management
- Provides health care to civilian government employees of the United States government

VI. MILITARY HEALTH INSURANCE

TRICARE

- Formerly known as CHAMPUS: Civilian Health and Medical Program of the Uniformed Services
- Program administered by the Department of Defense military health system for active duty and retired members and their dependents:
    - Uniformed services
    - National guard and reserve
    - Retired military and their families

CHAMPVA

- Civilian Health and Medical Program administered by the Department of Veterans Affairs
- Program in which the Veterans Administration shares the cost of covered health care services with spouses and unmarried children under the age of eighteen of veterans who have a 100 percent permanent disability

COORDINATION OF BENEFITS

Coordination of benefits is the process by which a health insurance company determines the order in which the insurance claim is paid when an individual is covered by more than one insurance plan. The health plan coordinates benefits with the other plan(s) to avoid duplicate payments to providers.

Payers

Primary payer: Pays for all eligible services
Secondary payer: Pays a portion or all remaining eligible charges not covered by the primary coverage

Determining Payers

Individuals covered under more than one plan:
- If the individual is covered under more than one employee plan, the plan that has been in effect the longest is primary
- When an individual is covered under one plan as an employee and under another as a dependent, the employee plan is primary, and the dependent plan is secondary

Children of divorced or separated parents:
- The plan of the custodial parent is primary
- If the custodial parent has remarried, then the plan of the spouse of the custodial parent is considered primary
- Lastly, the plan of the parent without custody is primary

Parents with joint custody:
- When parents share joint custody, the "Birthday Rule" will apply

Birthday Rule

The benefits for dependent children are determined under the plan of the parent whose birthday falls earliest in the year. For example, if the father's birthday is December 4 and mother's birthday is April 23, the dependent children would be covered under the plan of the mother since her birthday falls earlier in the year. This rule applies only to the birth month and day, not the year the parent was born.

MY KEY NOTES

PART IV

Medical Specialties

Specialists are physicians who have advanced training in a specific area of medicine. Classifications include:

Age-related specialties:

- Pediatrics: Birth through teens
- Family medicine: Infant through adulthood
- Internal medicine: Late teens through adulthood

Organ-related specialties:

- Gastroenterology: Stomach and intestines
- Nephrology: Kidneys
- Pulmonology: Lungs

Surgical specialties:

- Cardiovascular surgery: Heart and blood vessels
- Neurosurgery: Brain, spinal cord and nerves
- Thoracic surgery: Chest, ribs and lungs

ALLERGY & IMMUNOLOGY

ALLERGIST	Physician specializing in diagnosing and treating allergy symptoms, diseases, and disorders
IMMUNOLOGIST	Physician specializing in treating diseases and disorders of the immune system

KEY TERMS

Acquired immunity	Immunity that develops after exposure to an antigen
Allergen	Substance that causes an allergic response
Allergic response	Immune system overreacts and attacks a foreign substance that is normally harmless
Allergy	Hypersensitivity of the immune system in response to a foreign substance
Anaphylaxis	Severe allergic reaction and life-threatening condition
Antibody	Protein substance in the cell produced in response to an allergen
Antigen	Bacteria, virus, poison, or toxin that produces antibodies
Antihistamine	Medication that blocks the effect of histamine; reduces or prevents symptoms of an allergic response
Histamine	Protein compound involved in many allergic reactions
Immune response	Reaction of the immune system to a foreign substance
Immunity	Biological defense against foreign substances and toxins
Inflammatory response	Response of the body against disease or injury; injured body cells produce histamine that causes redness, heat, swelling, and pain

ALLERGY TESTS

Tests that check for the presence of specific antibodies and determine what substances trigger allergies:

- **Skin tests:**
    - Intradermal test   Small amount of an allergen is injected into the skin
    - Patch test   Allergen is applied to a patch that is then applied to the skin
    - Prick test   Small prick, puncture or scratch is made on the skin, and allergens are applied directly to the area
- **Blood tests:**
    - ELISA test   Enzyme-Linked Immunosorbent Assay
    - RAST test   Radioallergosorbent Test

ALLERGIC RESPONSE	
ALLERGENS • **FOOD** • **CHEMICAL** • **ENVIRONMENTAL**	Pollen Pet dander Food Mold Dust mites Chemicals
ENTER THE BODY	Skin contact Inhaled Swallowed Injected
ANTIBODIES	Attach to cells filled with histamine
HISTAMINE	Histamine causes cells to explode
SYMPTOMS	Allergic response occurs

IMMUNE SYSTEM

The immune system is the body's defense against disease-causing organisms and harmful substances (antigens). It tries to detect, destroy, and eliminate antigens before they enter the body and reproduce.

- The body creates barriers that keep antigens from entering:
    o Mucus
    o Saliva
    o Skin
    o Stomach acids
    o White blood cells
- Antibodies (protein substance produced in the cells) protect the body from antigens such as:
    o Bacteria
    o Fungi
    o Parasites
    o Toxins
    o Viruses

AUTOIMMUNE DISEASE

Autoimmune disease is a disorder where the body cannot distinguish between harmful substances and healthy body tissue.

- Chronic disabling condition in which the body attacks its own organs, tissues, and cells
- The body produces antibodies against its own normal healthy cells causing inflammation and injury
- There are over eighty autoimmune diseases including:
    o Anemia
    o Celiac disease
    o Crohn's disease
    o Inflammatory bowel disease
    o Leukemia
    o Lupus
    o Multiple sclerosis
    o Psoriasis
    o Rheumatoid arthritis
    o Type 1 Diabetes

Audiology

AUDIOLOGY	The study and treatment of hearing and balance disorders
AUDIOLOGIST	Individual specializing in diagnosing and treating hearing and balance problems

KEY TERMS

Acuity	Clarity, sharpness, keenness of perception
Audiogram	Chart showing a person's hearing ability over a range of frequencies
Audiometer	Instrument used to measure a person's hearing ability
Audiometry	Hearing test
Auditory canal	Tube leading into the middle ear
Auditory liquids	Watery liquids located in the cochlea that help conduct vibrations
Auditory nerve	Nerve that carries impulses from the cochlear to the brain; also known as the cochlear nerve or acoustic nerve
Auditory receptor cells	Hair-like cells that respond to vibrations
Cerumen	Waxy substance that lubricates the ear
Cochlea	Inner ear structure that picks up and carries sound
Ossicles	Bones located in the middle ear: hammer, anvil, and stirrup
Otoscope	Instrument with magnification and lighting features used to examine the ear
Tympanic membrane	Eardrum; membrane between the outer and middle ear that receives and transmits sound vibrations
TDD	Telecommunications Device for the Deaf

HEARING AIDS & COCHLEAR IMPLANTS

Hearing Aid

- Electronic device that amplifies sound
- Consists of a microphone, amplifier and receiver
- Worn in or around the ear
- Microphone picks up sounds and converts them into electrical signals
- Benefits people with mild to severe hearing loss

Cochlear Implant

- Prosthetic replacement for the inner ear (cochlea) that helps the hearing impaired to understand speech and recognize sound
  - Converts sounds into electrical impulses
  - Impulses stimulate hearing nerves
  - Brain interprets impulses as sound
- Electrodes are implanted in the ear, and a small device is worn on the body
- Appropriate for people with severe to profound hearing loss and who receive minimal or no benefit from a conventional hearing aid

SOUND

- Sound waves enter the ear and travel through the **auditory canal**

- Waves strike the **tympanic membrane** causing it to vibrate

- Vibration causes **ossicles** to move

- Movement carries sound waves to the **cochlea**

- Cochlea contains **auditory liquids,** which conduct vibrations

- Vibrations are received by **receptor cells,** and relay sound to the auditory nerve fibers

- **Auditory nerve fibers** transmit impulses to the brain where they are interpreted as **sound**

Cardiology

CARDIOLOGY	The study and treatment of heart disorders
CARDIOLOGIST	Physician specializing in diagnosing and treating heart disorders

KEY TERMS

Aneurysm	Widening of an artery
Angina	Chest pain and discomfort
Auscultation	Listening to the chest with a stethoscope for abnormal heart sounds
Blood vessels	Veins, arteries, and capillaries
Bradycardia	Slow heart rate
Cardiac surgeon	Physician specializing in open-heart surgery
Embolism	Obstruction of a blood vessel
Hypotension	Abnormally low blood pressure
Infarction	Sudden loss of blood supply
Ischemia	Inadequate blood supply
Lymph	Watery liquid that surrounds the cell
Occlusion	Blocked or closed passage
Sinus rhythm	Normal, regular heart beat
Stenosis	Narrowing of a blood vessel
Tachycardia	Fast heart rate
Thoracic surgeon	Physician who performs surgery on the heart, lungs, esophagus, and other organs of the chest
Vascular surgeon	Physician specializing in surgery on the vascular and lymphatic system

BLOOD PRESSURE (BP)

Blood pressure is the force or pressure of the blood inside the artery that is produced by the contraction and relaxation of the heart muscle.

- Blood pressure is recorded by two numbers and expressed as a fraction:

  120 = Systolic pressure
  80 = Diastolic pressure

  o Systolic pressure: Pressure during the beat when the heart muscle is contracting
  o Diastolic pressure: Pressure between beats when the heart is relaxing and refilling with blood

- Blood pressure is affected by:
  - Alcohol
  - Diet
  - Exercise
  - Heredity
  - Sleep patterns
  - Smoking
  - Stress levels

CIRCULATORY SYSTEMS

CIRCULATORY SYSTEM
- Heart and blood vessels
- Heart muscle pumps the blood, which travels through the blood vessels bringing nutrients to the cells

VASCULAR SYSTEM
- Blood vessels
- Blood vessels carry blood and lymph throughout the body, delivering oxygen and nutrients to the cells, and taking away waste products

LYMPHATIC SYSTEM
- Lymph capillaries, lymph vessels, lymph nodes, thymus gland, bone marrow, and spleen
- Assists with drainage, provides transportation for proteins and fats, and produces and stores cells to fight infection

CARDIAC CONDITIONS AND DISORDERS

Arrhythmia	Abnormal heart rhythms
Arteriosclerosis	Hardening and thickening of the artery walls
Atrial Fibrillation (AFIB)	Rapid and irregular heartbeat
Cerebrovascular Accident (CVA)	Stroke; blood flow to the brain is stopped or reduced
Congestive Heart Failure (CHF)	Heart pumps insufficient amount of blood
Coronary Artery Disease (CAD)	Blockage of arteries to the chest
Deep Vein Thrombosis (DVT)	Blood clot deep within a vein
Hypertension (HTN)	High blood pressure
Lymphedema	Swelling caused by excess fluid in the tissues
Myocardial Infarction (MI)	Heart attack; damage to the heart due to a sudden lack of oxygen
Peripheral Artery Disease (PAD)	Blockage of blood vessels outside of heart
Transient Ischemic Attack (TIA)	Mini-stroke; blood flow to the brain stops for a short time

CARDIAC TESTS AND PROCEDURES

Echocardiogram (ECHO)	Sound waves from an ultrasound are used to create images of the heart and surrounding area
Electrocardiogram (EKG/ECG)	Probes are placed on the patient's chest, and a machine measures the hearts electrical activity
Electrocardiogram Stress Test	Patient exercises on a treadmill or stationary bike as it increases in speed and elevation; heart rate, heart rhythm, and blood pressure are monitored
Holter Monitor	Small portable monitor (EKG) is worn around the patient's neck or waist usually for twenty-four to forty-eight hours to monitor the electrical activity of the heart

Chiropractic Medicine

CHIROPRACTIC MEDICINE	The study and treatment of injuries and disorders of the neck, back, and spine
CHIROPRACTOR	Health care professional who specializes in the treatment of injuries of the neck, back, and spine

KEY TERMS

Cavitation	Popping sound that occurs when a gas bubble containing oxygen, nitrogen, and carbon dioxide escapes from the joint fluid
Cervical	Pertaining to the neck
Coccyx	Tailbone
Dislocation	Separation of two bones where they meet at the joint
Lumbar	Pertaining to the lower back
Luxation	Complete dislocation
Manipulation	Quick, sudden, high velocity adjustment technique
Mobilization	Slow, low velocity adjustment technique
Sacral	Pertaining to the base of the spine
Subluxation	Incomplete or partial dislocation
Thoracic	Pertaining to the chest

CHIROPRACTIC MEDICINE

Chiropractic medicine is a natural method of health care. It focuses on the cause of illness, injury, and disease, not just treating the symptoms. It is based on the fact that your body is able to heal itself when the spine and nervous systems are healthy and functioning properly.

CHIROPRACTORS
- Treat disorders without drugs or surgery
- Utilize techniques such as touch, massage, manipulation, and mobilization
- Believe that misalignment of the spine puts pressure on parts of the nervous system and lowers resistance to disease
- Acknowledge that many factors, including exercise, diet, and sleep contribute to overall health
- Trust in the body's natural ability to heal itself

SPINE
- Also known as the backbone, spinal or vertebral column
- Provides support for the body and protects the spinal cord
- Consists of individual bones that interlock to form the spinal column
- Divided into five sections

SPINE		
Cervical	Neck	Supports the weight of the head
Thoracic	Upper and middle back	Protects the organs of the chest
Lumbar	Lower back	Supports the weight of the body
Sacral	Base of the spine	Protects the pelvic organs
Coccyx	Tailbone	No recognized function

Dermatology

DERMATOLOGY	The study and treatment of the skin, hair, and nail diseases and disorders
DERMATOLOGIST	Physician specializing in the diagnosis and treatment of skin, hair, and nail diseases and disorders

KEY TERMS

Collagen	Protein in the connective tissue that provides strength
Elastin	Protein in the connective tissue that provides elasticity
Melanin	Pigment that gives skin, eye, and hair color

SKIN	
Protection	Protects from loss of: • Heat • Salt • Water
Secretion	Sebaceous glands: Produce an oily substance called sebum for lubrication Sweat glands: Produce a watery substance called sweat to cool the body
Regulation	Contains receptors for pain, touch, and pressure Carry impulses to the brain to regulate body temperature

SKIN CANCER

Melanoma
- Can appear on any part of the body
- Develops in cells that make pigment that gives skin its color

Non-Melanoma
- Basal and squamous cell carcinoma
- Develops mainly on the parts of the body exposed to the sun

American Cancer Society's ABCD RULE		
	NORMAL MOLE	**MELANOMA MOLE**
Asymmetry	Symmetrical	Not symmetrical
Border	Distinct border	Uneven, notched border
Color	One color	Mixture of several colors
Diameter	Less than six mm wide	More than six mm wide

SKIN CONDITIONS AND DISORDERS

Acne	Chronic skin condition with increased production of sebum, pimples, and inflammation
Cellulitis	Bacterial infection of the deeper layers of the skin causing redness and itching
Dermatitis	Skin conditions characterized by inflammation, redness, and itching
Eczema	Inflammatory rash with redness, swelling, bumps, and itching
Impetigo	Bacterial infection characterized by blisters, pustules, and lesions
Psoriasis	Chronic, recurrent skin condition characterized by red, itchy, and scaly patches
Rosacea	Chronic condition marked by persistent redness of the skin
Seborrhea	Dandruff; thick, flaky patches of scale on the head
Urticaria	Skin rash with red or white, raised, and itchy bumps; hives
Vitiligo	Disorder that causes loss of pigment in the skin

Endocrinology

ENDOCRINOLOGY	The study and treatment of the endocrine glands and the hormones they secrete
ENDOCRINOLOGIST	Physician specializing in the treatment, diagnosis, and management of endocrine disease and disorders

KEY TERMS

Blood sugar	Amount of glucose present in the blood
Gland	Group of cells that secrete a substance for use in the body, or that remove harmful materials from the blood
Glucose	Simple sugar; main energy source for the body
Hormone	Chemical substance produced by the body that regulates the activity of specific cells and organs
Insulin	Hormone secreted by the pancreas gland that controls the level of glucose in the blood
Metabolism	Process of breaking down food and converting it into energy

ENDOCRINE SYSTEM

Main body system for communication and coordination. The endocrine system works with the nervous system, reproductive system, kidneys, pancreas, and liver to control:

- Energy levels
- Equilibrium of internal body systems
- Growth and development
- Production, storage, and release of hormones
- Response to stress and injury

ENDOCRINE GLANDS

Adrenal	Regulates salt, heart rate, and blood pressure
Hypothalamus	Controls temperature, hunger, thirst, and behavior
Ovaries	Secretes female reproductive hormones
Pancreas	Produces insulin and regulates blood sugar levels
Parathyroid	Regulates calcium level in the blood
Pineal	Controls sleep and mood
Pituitary	Links the endocrine system and nervous systems
Testes	Secretes male reproductive hormones
Thymus	Necessary for the immune function in newborns
Thyroid	Regulates metabolism and growth

ENDOCRINE CONDITIONS AND DISORDERS

Hyperglycemia	High glucose levels in the blood
Hyperlipidemia	High cholesterol levels in the blood
Hyperthyroidism	Overactive thyroid, fast metabolism
Hypoglycemia	Low glucose levels in the blood
Hypolipidemia	Low blood cholesterol levels
Hypothyroidism	Underactive thyroid, slow metabolism

Diabetes:

Gestational Diabetes:
- Diabetic symptoms that appear during pregnancy

Type 1 Diabetes:
- Body does not produce insulin
- Previously known as Insulin-dependent diabetes mellitus

Type 2 Diabetes:
- Body produces a small amount of insulin
- Previously known as non-insulin dependent diabetes mellitus

TYPE 2 DIABETES	
Healthy Individual	• Glucose and insulin are present during digestion • Insulin "unlocks" cells so glucose can enter • Energy is produced
Type 2 Diabetic	• Body does not produce enough insulin • Glucose is "locked out" of the cell when not enough insulin is present • Blood sugar rises

Gastroenterology

GASTROENTEROLOGY	The study and treatment of digestive system diseases and disorders
GASTROENTEROLOGIST	Physician specializing in the diagnosis, treatment, and management of diseases and disorders of the digestive system

KEY TERMS

Absorption	Process by which substances enter the bloodstream during digestion
Barium	Substance administered to patients before x-rays of the gastrointestinal tract are taken; provides visibility of the organs
Bile	Digestive fluid that breaks down fat
Defecation	Elimination of feces through the rectum
Deglutition	Swallowing
Digestion	Process of breaking down substances for energy and growth
Elimination	Process of discharging waste products from the body
Enzymes	Chemical that speeds up the reaction between two substances
Gastric	Pertaining to the stomach
Mastication	Process by which food is ground by the teeth; chewing
Motility	Movement of food through the stomach and intestine
Nutrients	Final by-products of digestion that are reabsorbed
Peristalsis	Involuntary contraction of the muscles

ORAL CAVITY

Where: Teeth, tongue, gums, and tonsils

What: Food is chewed and broken down with the enzymes in the saliva.

How: Mastication (chewing)
Deglutition (swallowing)

UPPER GASTROINTESTINAL TRACT

Where: Pharynx, esophagus, and stomach

What: Pharynx serves as a passageway for food to the esophagus where the process of peristalsis begins. Food then passes to the stomach where it is broken down further with the help of the enzyme pepsin.

How: Deglutition (swallowing)
Peristalsis (contraction)
Motility (movement)

LOWER GASTROINTESTINAL TRACT

Where: Small intestine, liver, gallbladder, pancreas, large intestine, and rectum

What: Food passes into the small intestine and is broken down with the help of pancreatic enzymes and bile. Large intestine absorbs most of the water from the waste products of digestion. Body eliminates waste products in the form of feces.

How: Peristalsis (contraction)
Motility (movement)
Defecation (elimination)

GASTROINTESTINAL CONDITIONS AND DISORDERS

Celiac Disease	Inability of the body to absorb certain nutrients; damage to the small intestine due to gluten intolerance
Cirrhosis	Scarring of the liver and poor liver function
Colitis	Inflammation of the large intestine
Diverticulitis	Inflamed pouch pockets in the lining of the abdominal wall
Dysphagia	Difficulty swallowing
Hepatitis	Inflammation of the liver

Inflammatory Bowel Disease (IBD)
- Crohn's Disease: Inflammation of the intestinal tract
- Ulcerative Colitis   Inflammation of the large intestine

Irritable Bowel Syndrome (IBS)
- Constipation   Infrequent, difficult bowel movement
- Diarrhea   Loose, watery bowel movements

Peptic Ulcer Disease (PUD)   Open sores in the digestive tract
- Duodenal ulcers   Sores that occur in the small intestine
- Esophageal ulcers   Sores that occur in the esophagus
- Gastric ulcers   Sores that occur in the stomach

GASTROESOPHAGEAL REFLUX DISEASE (GERD)

Recurrent disorder where the acidic stomach contents flow back up (reflux) into the esophagus:
- A sphincter muscle connects the esophagus to the stomach
- This muscle works as a gate, allowing food in and then closing again
- People with GERD have a sphincter (gate) that does not work properly
- Stomach contents reflux into the esophagus, causing inflammation, pain, and discomfort

ENDOCSCOPY

An endoscopy is an examination of the internal structures using an instrument called an endoscope. It is a thin, flexible, lighted tube with a tiny camera attached. Some procedures incorporate other attachments such as probes, cutting tools and electric current. Entry is made through the mouth, anus or an incision. Endoscopic procedures are used to:

- Diagnose and monitor medical conditions
- Treat disease
- Provide visual evidence
- Acquire tissue specimens
- Obtain photographs
- Perform procedures

Considered minimally invasive surgery, multiple endoscopic procedures have been developed for different parts of the body. Procedures performed on the gastrointestinal tract include:

• Colonoscopy	Large intestine
• Enteroscopy	Small intestine
• Esophagoscopy	Esophagus
• Gastroscopy	Stomach
• Laparoscopy	Abdominal organs
• Sigmoidoscopy	Colon
• Upper Endoscopy	Esophagus, stomach, and small intestine

GASTROINTESTINAL TESTS AND PROCEDURES

Barium Enema	Colon is filled with barium liquid (contrast medium), and then a series of x-rays are taken of the colon and rectum; also known as a Lower GI Series
Barium Swallow	Patient drinks barium liquid, and then a series of x-rays are taken of the esophagus, stomach, and small intestine; also known as an Upper GI Series
Fecal Occult Blood Test	Lab test that checks for hidden blood in stool that may indicate disease
Liver Biopsy	Specimen from the liver is removed and examined under a microscope for damage or disease

Hematology

HEMATOLOGY	The study and treatment of blood, blood diseases, and the blood-forming organs
HEMATOLOGIST	Physician specializing in the diagnosis and treatment of diseases and disorders of the blood and blood-forming organs

KEY TERMS

Aplasia	Incomplete or defective development
Bleeding time	Time required for a small standard wound to stop bleeding
Blood	Body fluid that provides nutrients and oxygen to the cells and carries away waste products
Blood organs	Organs that make blood cells
Cells	Smallest unit of life
Coagulation time	Time required for blood to clot under controlled conditions
Erythrocytes	Red blood cells; deliver oxygen to the tissues
Hematocrit	Percentage of blood volume that is made up of red blood cells
Hemoglobin	Protein in red blood cells
Leukocytes	White blood cells; defend against infection
Organs	Collection of tissues working together for a common purpose
Plasma	Liquid portion of the blood containing water, proteins, vitamins, and nutrients
Platelets	Blood component that assists with clotting and the repair of damaged tissue
Tissues	Collection of cells working together for a common function

BLOOD SYSTEM

The blood is made up of three main components, cells, platelets and, plasma and:

- Carries nutrients
- Transports oxygen
- Directs hormones
- Removes waste products
- Regulates body temperature
- Assists with clotting

ANEMIA

Deficiency of red blood cells or low in hemoglobin caused by:

Insufficient or decreased production of red blood cells

- Iron deficiency
- Vitamin deficiency anemia

Destruction of red blood cells

- Sickle cell anemia
- Thalassemia

Loss of blood through bleeding

- Gastrointestinal conditions such as ulcers
- Menstruation
- Childbirth

BLOOD CONDITIONS AND DISORDERS

Blood dyscrasia	Diseases of the blood and blood-forming organs
Hemophilia	Genetic disorder where the blood does not clot properly, resulting in excessive bleeding
Sepsis	Life-threatening infection of the blood and blood-forming organs
Thrombosis	Blood clot in a blood vessel that obstructs blood flow
Von Willebrand Disease	Disorder where blood does not clot properly

Infectious Disease (ID)

INFECTIOUS DISEASE	Disease caused by contact with bacteria, virus, fungus, or parasites
ID SPECIALIST	Physician of internal medicine who specializes in the diagnosis and treatment of infectious disease

KEY TERMS

Epidemic Sudden outbreak of an illness or health-related issue that shows up in more cases than expected in a community; outbreak covers a small geographic area.

Pandemic Outbreak of an illness usually caused by a new strain of virus that most people have little resistance to; outbreak covers a large geographic area.

TYPES OF INFECTIONS AND DISEASE

Bacterial: Infection and disease caused by bacteria

- Chlamydia
- E. Coli
- Lyme Disease
- Pertussis
- Staphylococcus
- Streptococcus
- Syphilis
- Tuberculosis

Viral: Infection and disease caused by a virus

- AIDS
- Chicken Pox
- Hepatitis A, B, C
- HIV
- HPV
- Influenza
- Measles
- Mononucleosis
- Mumps
- Rubella
- Upper Respiratory Infection (URI)

Fungal: Infection and disease caused by fungus

- Athlete's foot
- Candida
- Ringworm
- Thrush

Parasitic: Infection and disease caused by parasites

- Malaria
- Scabies

TRANSMISSION OF INFECTIOUS DISEASE

- Inhaling airborne germs
- Ingesting contaminated food or water
- Insect or animal bite
- Person-to-person contact via:
  - Blood
  - Cough
  - Kiss
  - Mother to infant
  - Sex
  - Skin
  - Sneeze

HIV and AIDS

HIV (Human Immunodeficiency Virus) is the **VIRUS** that causes AIDS (Acquired Immune Deficiency Syndrome) the **DISEASE**

OPPORTUNISTIC INFECTIONS

- Type of infection that occurs because of an already weakened immune system
- Often associated with AIDS because it lowers resistance and allows infections that a healthy immune system could contain

STAGES OF HIV/AIDS	
Window	Period between time of infection and symptoms
Acute Infection	Large amounts of virus are produced Flu-like symptoms are present
Latency Period	Virus is producing at very low levels No symptoms are present
AIDS	T-cell (type of white blood cell) count is below two hundred Opportunistic infections are present

Laboratory and Pathology

LABORATORY	A place equipped to conduct scientific tests and experiments
PATHOLOGY	The study of disease and the examination and analysis of tissue and organs for diagnosis

KEY TERMS

Biopsy	Removal of a tissue sample for examination
Culture	Growth of microorganisms or viruses for identification purposes and study
Phlebotomy	Obtaining blood from a vein
Specimen	Sample of a substance or material for examination and study

SPECIMEN COLLECTION

Blood	**Venipuncture:** Obtaining blood from a vein using a needle
Urine	**Urinalysis:** Collection of urine directly into a sterile container
Biopsy	**Needle Biopsy:** Cells and tissue are withdrawn using a syringe **Open Biopsy:** Incision is made and tissue is cut from site
Phlegm	**Swab:** Samples are obtained using a swab **Expectorate:** Coughing up and spitting out phlegm into a sterile container
Stool	**Sample:** Collection of stool directly into a sterile container

ROUTINE BLOOD TESTS

Complete Blood Count (CBC)
- Group of tests that evaluate overall health

- Detect infections, clotting problems, cancers, and immune system disorders

Red Blood Cells

White Blood Cells

Platelets

Hemoglobin

Hematocrit

Mean Corpuscular Volume

Basic Metabolic Panel (BMP)
- Group of tests that measure chemicals in the blood

- Provide information on the heart, kidneys, liver, muscles, and bones

- Also known as Blood Chemistry Tests

Blood Glucose

Calcium

Electrolytes

Blood Urea Nitrogen

Creatinine

Blood Enzyme Tests
- Tests for heart attack by checking levels of the enzymes released in response to heart damage

Troponin

Creatine Kinase

Lipid Panel
- Tests that determine your risk for coronary disease

- Also known as Lipid Profile and Coronary Risk Panel

Total Cholesterol

LDL "bad" Cholesterol

HDL "good" Cholesterol

Triglycerides

Nephrology

NEPHROLOGY	The study and treatment of diseases and disorders of the kidneys
NEPHROLOGIST	Physician specializing in the diagnosis and treatment of kidney diseases and disorders

KEY TERMS

Filtration	Process of separating materials using a filter
Reabsorption	Process by which the necessary materials and nutrients are returned to the bloodstream

KIDNEYS

The kidneys are a pair of bean-shaped organs located just below the ribs on either side of the spine that:

- Balance fluid and mineral levels
- Filter blood
- Remove waste products
- Help control blood pressure
- Release hormones
- Regulate electrolytes

EXCRETION AND SECRETION

Excretion

- Removal of material from an organism
  - Sweat: Released through the skin
  - Carbon dioxide: Exhaled from the lungs
  - Metabolic waste: Excreted in urine
  - Undigested food: Excreted in bowel movements

Secretion

- Movement of material for one place to another
  - Salvia
  - Enzymes
  - Hormones

DIALYSIS

Dialysis performs the work of a failed kidney by getting rid of excess fluid, and separating nutrients and waste products from the blood.

Hemodialysis

- Filtering machine, also know as an artificial kidney, receives waste-filled blood from the patient's body, filters it, and returns nutrient rich blood back into the bloodstream

Peritoneal Dialysis

- Permanent tube introduces fluid into the abdominal cavity
- Chemicals in the fluid cause the waste products in the blood to pass out of the bloodstream
- Membrane in the abdominal cavity acts as a filter
- Nutrients remain in the blood and waste products are removed

KIDNEY CONDITIONS AND DISORDERS

Chronic Kidney Disease (CKD)	Progressive loss of kidney function
Chronic Renal Failure (CRF)	Kidney Failure
End Stage Renal Disease (ESRD)	Failure of kidneys to function on their own
Polycystic Kidney Disease (PKD)	Genetic disorder characterized by the growth of fluid filled cysts in and on the kidney
Urinary stones:	Hard build up of minerals
• **Nephrolithiasis**	Kidney stones
• **Cystolithiasis**	Bladder stones
• **Ureterolithiasis**	Ureter stones

KIDNEY TESTS

Glomerular Filtration Rate (GFR)	Measures the ability of the kidneys to filter and remove toxins and waste products
Kidney Function Tests (KFT)	Collective term for a variety of blood and urine tests which measure and evaluate kidney function

Neurology

NEUROLOGY	The study and treatment of nervous system disorders
NEUROLOGIST	Physician specializing in the diagnosis and treatment of nervous system disorders

KEY TERMS

Genetic
- Pertaining to genes and heredity

Congenital
- Present at birth
- Result of factors that occur while the fetus is still in-utero
- Not a result of family history or genetics

Hereditary
- Genetically predetermined
- Dependent on inherited genes passed to the fetus from the father and the mother

NERVOUS SYSTEM

- Regulates temperature, blood pressure, heart rate, and breathing
- Processes information received through the senses
- Coordinates movement and motion
- Assists with reasoning, feelings, and emotions
- Consists of two systems
    - Central Nervous System (CNS): Brain and spinal cord
    - Peripheral Nervous System (PNS): Nerves

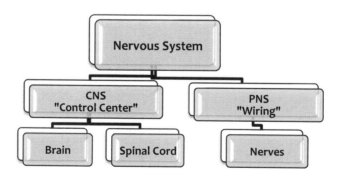

PARTS OF THE BRAIN

- Brain stem   Controls heartbeat and breathing
- Cerebellum   Coordinates balance and movement
- Cerebrum   Controls thinking and voluntary muscles
- Hypothalamus   Regulates temperature
- Pituitary gland   Controls growth
- Thalamus   Relays messages and transmits replies

NEUROLOGICAL CONDITIONS AND DISORDERS

Alzheimer's Disease	Degenerative disorder that causes irreversible and progressive loss of mental function
Autism	Developmental disorder causing delayed language development, trouble with social interactions, and sensory overload
Cerebral Palsy	Developmental disorder affecting learning, movement, and coordination
Epilepsy	Disorder characterized by repeated seizures
Multiple Sclerosis	Chronic and inflammatory disease of the brain and spinal cord characterized by fatigue, numbness, and balance and coordination problems
Parkinson's Disease	Movement and degenerative disorder causing rigid muscles, tremors, and difficulty with speech

NEUROLOGICAL TESTS AND PROCEDURES

Cerebrospinal Fluid Analysis (CSF)	Laboratory test on spinal fluid to diagnose CNS conditions
Electroencephalogram (EEG)	Records the electrical activity of the brain and detects abnormalities
Electromyography (EMG)	Measures the muscle response and electrical activity after stimulation of a nerve
Electronystagmography (ENG)	Group of radiology tests to diagnosis balance disorders
Myelogram	Radiology procedure to evaluate the spinal cord, nerves, and tissues
Nerve Conduction Velocity (NCV)	Measures the speed conduction of an impulse through the nerve

Obstetrics and Gynecology OB/GYN

OBSTETRICS/GYN	The study and treatment of the conditions and diseases of the female reproductive system, including hormones and breasts
OBSTETRICIAN/GYN	Physician specializing in the diagnosis and treatment of conditions of the female reproductive system

KEY TERMS

Estrogen	Hormone responsible for female secondary sex characteristics
Menopause	Cessation of menstruation; diminished hormone production
Menstruation	Onset of puberty; shedding of the uterine lining and bleeding
Ovary	Female sex hormone; secretes estrogen and progesterone
Progesterone	Hormone responsible for menstrual cycle

OBSTETRIC AND GYNECOLOGICAL CONDITIONS

Ectopic Pregnancy	Embedding of the fertilized egg outside of the uterus
Endometriosis	Cells from the uterus grow in other parts of the body causing pain, bleeding, and fertility problems
Fibrocystic Breast	Non-cancerous condition causing lumpy and painful breasts
Fibroids	Non-cancerous tumors in the uterus
Infertility	Inability to become pregnant
Ovarian Cysts	Fluid-filled sacs located in the ovaries
Pelvic Inflammatory Disease	Inflammation and infection of the reproductive organs
Pregnancy	Uterus containing a developing fetus
Premenstrual Syndrome	Range of symptoms that start prior to a woman's period

Oncology

ONCOLOGY	The study and treatment of cancer
ONCOLOGIST	Physician specializing in the diagnosis and treatment of cancer

KEY TERMS

Benign	Non-cancerous; not invading nearby tissue or spreading
Cancer	Disease caused by an abnormal and excessive growth of cells in the body
Carcinogenesis	Transformation of a normal cell into a cancerous cell
Carcinoma	Cancer located in the epithelial tissue
Dysplasia	Abnormal change in size and shape in a group of cells
Hyperplasia	Overgrowth of cells in a specific tissue
In Situ	Cancer is confined to a particular area and has not spread
Leukemia	Cancer located in the blood-forming tissue
Lymphoma	Cancer located in the lymphoid tissue
Malignant	Cancerous; capable of invasion and spread to other sites
Metastasis	Spread of a malignant tumor to a secondary site
Neoplasms	Tumors; masses or growths that arise from normal tissue
Sarcoma	Cancer located in the connective tissue
Staging	Process of determining how far a cancer has spread
Tumor	Abnormal enlargement of cells or tissues

CANCER

- Broad group of diseases characterized by cells that divide, grow, and replicate at an alarming and uncontrolled rate
- Can develop in most organs and tissues
- Always named after the place it started

CANCER	

Carcinoma	• Tumors located in the epithelial tissue
	• Epithelial tissue lines the external surfaces and internal structures: digestive organs, glands, reproductive organs, skin, urinary organs:
	   o Bladder
	   o Breast
	   o Colon
	   o Kidney
	   o Stomach
	   o Lung
	   o Liver
	   o Prostate

Sarcoma	• Tumors located in the connective tissue
	• Connective tissue serves as structure and support:
	   o Fat
	   o Bone
	   o Muscle
	   o Cartilage
	   o Blood vessels

Lymphoma	• Tumors located in the lymph nodes and tissues of the body's immune system
	   o Hodgkin's
	   o Non-Hodgkin's

Leukemia	• Cancer of the cells that grow in the bone marrow and accumulate in the blood and blood-forming organs.

Ophthalmology

OPHTHALMOLOGY	The study and treatment of eye diseases and disorders
OPHTHALMOLOGIST	Physician specializing in the diagnosis and treatment of eye diseases and disorders

KEY TERMS

Optician   Professional who designs, fits, and dispenses eyeglasses and contact lenses

Optometrists   Practitioner who performs eye exams, treats vision problems, writes prescriptions

PARTS OF THE EYE	
Cornea	Transparent dome on the outer part of the eye that focuses light
Iris	Colored part of the eye that regulates the amount of light entering
Lens	Clear part of the eye that helps refract and focus light
Macula	Area of the retina that gives vision
Optic Nerve	Nerves that carry visual signals from the retina to the brain
Pupil	Black circle in the center of the eye through which light passes
Retina	Membrane that acts as a screen, changing light into nerve signals
Sclera	White part of the eye that covers the eyeball
Vitreous Body	Clear, gel-like lubricating substance

EYE CONDITIONS AND DISORDERS

Astigmatism	Imperfection in the curvature of the cornea
Blepharitis	Inflammation of the eyelid
Cataract	Cloudy area in the normally clear lens of the eye that obstructs the passage of light
Color Blindness	Cannot distinguish between certain colors
Conjunctivitis	Pink eye; swelling of the membrane of the eye
Corneal Abrasion	Scratch on the cornea, causing severe pain and inflammation
Corneal Laceration	Cut on the cornea, causing severe pain and inflammation
Detached Retina	Separation of the layers of the retina; retina pulls away from the back of the eye
Glaucoma	Build up in eye pressure that results in optic nerve damage and loss of vision
Hyperopia	Farsightedness; distant objects are seen clearly
Macular Degeneration	Progressive damage to the macula of the retina, resulting in loss of central vision
Myopia	Nearsightedness; nearby objects are seen clearly

EYE TESTS AND PROCEDURES

Dilation Test	Drops are placed into the eyes to make the pupils larger in order to gain a better view of the internal eye structures
Glaucoma Test	Measures the pressure inside of the eye
Refraction Test	Eye chart is read at a distance of twenty feet; determines eyeglass prescription
Slit Lamp Exam	Provides a three-dimensional view of the interior of the eye
Visual Field Test	Measures scope of central and peripheral vision

Orthopedics

ORTHOPEDICS	The study of diseases and disorders of the bones, muscles, and joints
ORTHOPEDIST	Physician specializing in the diagnosis and disorders of the bones, muscles, and joints

KEY TERMS

Cartilage	Firm, rubbery tissue that cushions the bones
Disc	Spongy, cushion-like pads between the vertebrae
Joint	Point where two bones interconnect
Fracture	Breaking of a bone
• Incomplete	One break in a bone
• Complete	Two or more breaks in a bone
• Simple	Skin covering the bone is undamaged
• Compound	Surface of the skin tears and the bone is exposed
Ligament	Connective tissue that connects bone to bone
Tendon	Connective tissue that connects muscle to bone
Vertebrae	Individual bones of the spine
Vertebrate	Backbone

MUSCULOSKELETAL SYSTEM

Bones: Provide protection and framework for the body

• Long	Legs
• Short	Wrist
• Flat	Ribs
• Sesamoid	Kneecap

Muscles: Provide movement

• Skeletal	Voluntary
• Smooth	Involuntary
• Cardiac	Heart

Joints: Provide flexibility

• Synovial	Moveable
• Suture	Immovable

MAJOR BONES OF THE BODY

Cranium:	Scull	Phalanges:	Fingers
Maxilla:	Upper jaw	Metacarpals:	Hand bones
Mandible:	Lower jaw	Pelvis:	Hip
Clavicle:	Collarbone	Vertebrate:	Backbone
Scapula:	Shoulder blade	Femur:	Thighbone
Sternum:	Breastbone	Patella:	Kneecap
Humorous:	Upper arm bone	Fibula:	Small, lower leg
Radius:	Inner, lower arm	Tibia:	Large, lower leg
Ulna:	Outer, lower arm	Tarsal:	Ankle
Carpals:	Wrist	Phalanges:	Toes

ORTHOPEDIC CONDITIONS & DISORDERS

Arthritis	Inflammation of the joints
Bursitis	Inflammation of the bursa
Carpal Tunnel	Pressure on the nerve causing numbness and pain
Cartilage Injuries	Injury to the tissue that cushions the bones
Dislocations	Separation of bones at the joint
Fractures	Breaking of a bone
Ligament Injuries	Injury to the tissue surrounding the joint
Osteomyelitis	Infection of the bone
Osteoporosis	Loss of bone density
Scoliosis	Abnormal curving of the spine
Sprains	Trauma to joints or ligaments
Strains	Overstretching or tearing of a muscle
Tendonitis	Inflammation of the tendon

ORTHOPEDIC TESTS AND PROCEDURES

Arthrography	Series of x-rays of a joint, using contrast medium, to diagnose the cause of unexplained joint pain
Arthroplasty	Replacement of a joint, such a hip or knee, using an artificial prosthesis
Arthroscopy	Examination of a joint through a small incision using a flexible, viewing device
Bone Density	Radiology test that measures bone mineral content
Bone Scan	Nuclear test to diagnose inflammation, cancer or abnormal bone growth

Otolaryngology / ENT

OTOLARYNGOLOGIST	The study and treatment of diseases and disorders of the ears, nose, throat, head, and neck
OTOLARYNGOLOGIST	Physician specializing in the diagnosis and treatment of diseases and disorders of the ears, nose, throat, head, and neck

KEY TERMS

Epiglottis   Small flap-like structure that closes over the larynx

Larynx   Voice box

Pharynx   Throat

Tonsil   Lymph tissue located in the back of the mouth

Trachea   Windpipe

Ear: Treatment for hearing disorders, balance problems, and infections
- Otitis Externa   Infection/inflammation of the outer ear
- Otitis Media   Infection/inflammation of the middle ear
- Tinnitus   Abnormal ringing in the ears
- Vertigo   Dizziness; sensation of a whirling motion

Nose: Treatment of the nasal cavity and sinuses
- Allergy   Hypersensitivity of the immune system
- Rhinitis   Inflammation/irritation of the nose
- Sinusitis   Inflammation/irritation of the sinuses

Throat: Treatment for disease of the larynx and swallowing disorders
- Laryngitis   Inflammation/irritation of the vocal cords
- Pharyngitis   Inflammation/irritation of the throat
- Tonsillitis   Inflammation/irritation of the tonsils
- Dysphagia   Difficulty swallowing

Head and neck: Treatment for disease; surgery
- Injectable fillers
- Plastic surgery
- Reconstructive surgery
- Tumors

Pain Management

PAIN MANAGEMENT	Discipline concerned with pain
PAIN SPECIALIST	Physician specializing in pain management

KEY TERMS

Acute Pain	Sudden onset; lasts a short time
Chronic Pain	Slow onset; lasts several months or more
Nerve Pain	Pain located within the nervous system
Somatic Pain	Pain located in the skin, bones, muscles, and ligaments
Visceral Pain	Pain located in the internal organs

PAIN ASSESSMENT

• Location	Where the pain is located
• Frequency	How often the pain occurs
• Description	Sharp, burning, stabbing, throbbing
• Intensity	Measured using a pain scale

PAIN SCALES

Pain scales measure the intensity of a patient's pain:

• Numerical	Scale from zero to ten - zero is no pain, and ten is severe pain
• Verbal	Patients respond verbally, describing their pain level by using the word no pain, mild pain, moderate pain, or severe pain
• Visual	Patients put a mark on a horizontal line indicating their level of pain

PAIN MANAGEMENT CONTRACT

Physicians often require that patients sign a pain contract as a condition of care for chronic pain. These agreements are commonly used when narcotics are prescribed. A pain management contract may include the flowing conditions:

- Patient must comply with all scheduled appointments
- Patient must agree not to receive any additional controlled substances from any other source or provider
- Lost or stolen prescriptions will not be replaced
- Patient must consent to random drug testing

Pharmacology

PHARMACOLOGY	The study of the preparations, properties, uses, and actions of drugs
PHARMACOLOGIST	Specialist concentrating in the research, development and testing of drugs for medical use
PHARMACIST	Professional who dispenses medication and educates individuals on their use

KEY TERMS

Brand Name Drug	Prescription drug that has been researched, developed, and manufactured by a pharmaceutical company and is patent protected for a period of time
Chemical Name Drug	Scientific name; specifies the chemical makeup of the drug
Formulary Drug	List of medications covered under a health insurance plan; usually include brand name and generic drugs
Generic Name Drug	Duplicate or twin of a name brand drug; once a brand name patent has expired, other companies may copy and manufacture it; it is less expensive because the company distributing it did not have to pay for the research and development
Non-formulary Drug	Drugs that have not yet been reviewed for formulary status

ROUTES OF ADMINISTERING MEDICINE

- Inhalation   Vapors or gases taken in by nose or mouth
- Oral   By mouth
- Parenteral   Injection of drugs from a syringe
- Rectal   Placed into the rectum
- Sublingual   Placed under the tongue
- Topical   Applied directly to skin

DRUG CATEGORIES	
Analgesics	Lessen pain
Anesthetics	Reduce or eliminate sensation
Antibiotics	Kill bacteria
Anticoagulants	Break up existing clots and prevent more from forming
Antidepressants	Elevate mood
Antihistamines	Block histamine
Antiplatelets	Reduce the tendency of blood platelets to stick together
Antivirals	Kill virus
Sedatives	Suppress the central nervous system; promote sleep
Stimulants	Act on the brain to speed up the vital processes
Tranquilizers	Control anxiety

CONTROLLED SUBSTANCES ACT

The Controlled Substances Act of 1970 classified drugs onto five schedules, according to their potential for abuse and dependence. The schedules range from I (most restricted) to V (least restricted).

SCHEDULE I
- High level for abuse
- These substances cannot be used for any purposes except medical research
- No prescription may be written on Schedule I substances
- Examples: heroin, LSD

SCHEDULE II
- Abuse may lead to severe psychological and physical dependence
- Prescription must be in writing and limited to a thirty-day supply (some exceptions)
- Prescriptions cannot be phoned into the pharmacy; a written prescription (Rx) must be presented to the pharmacist
- Examples: opium, morphine

SCHEDULE III
- Abuse may lead to low or moderate physical and psychological dependence
- Substances in this class require new written prescriptions after six months or five refills
- Examples: amphetamines, barbiturates, and anabolic steroids

SCHEDULE IV
- Abuse may lead to limited physical and psychological dependence
- Prescriptions must be written and may be refilled up to five times in a six-month period
- Examples: alprazolam, clonazepam, diazepam

SCHEDULE V
- Abuse may lead to some physical and psychological dependence
- This class is least restrictive
- Includes any non-narcotic prescription drugs and drugs that may be dispensed without a prescription

PHARMACEUTICAL ABBREVIATIONS

a.c. / ac	before meals
ad lib	freely, as desired
aq.	water
bid	twice a day
caps	capsules
da / daw	dispense as written
gtt.	drops
h.	hour
hs	at bedtime
NPO	nothing by mouth
pc	after meals
po / PO	by mouth
PRN	as needed
q	every day
qAM	every morning
qPM	every evening
q.d.	once a day
qh	every hour
qid	four times a day
q2h	every two hours
q3h	every three hours
q4h	every four hours
Sig	directions
s.o.s.	if necessary
stat.	immediately
tab	tablet
tid	three times a day
ut dict	as directed

Physical Therapy (PT)

PHYSICAL THERAPY	Treatment of disorders of the bones, muscles and joints, as well as stroke, arthritis, and brain and nerve conditions through physical means, manual therapy, and exercise
PHYSICAL THERAPIST	Health care professional specializing in rehabilitation

KEY TERMS

Active Exercise	Any exercise where the patient uses his or her own muscle strength
Isometric Exercise	Passive exercises done from a stationary position
Isotonic Exercise	Active exercises such as resistance or weight training
Passive Exercise	Any exercise technique performed on the patient by a therapist
Range of Motion	Distance and direction a joint can move to its full ability or potential

TYPES OF PHYSICAL THERAPY

Cardiovascular PT	Focuses on patients with heart and lung problems to improve strength and endurance
Geriatric PT	Works with senior citizens suffering from arthritis, osteoporosis, and joint replacement therapy to restore mobility
Neurological PT	Teaches patients with brain injuries how to improve and restore function
Orthopedic PT	Rehabilitation for disorders of the musculoskeletal system after surgery, accident, or injury

PT THERAPIES

- Electrical stimulation
- Exercise
- Hydrotherapy
- Massage
- Paraffin baths
- Heat treatment
- Cold treatments
- Traction

Podiatry

PODIATRY	The study and treatment of diseases, disorders, and deformities of the foot
PODIATRIST	Physician specializing in the diagnosis and treatment of foot disease, disorders, and deformities

KEY TERMS

Gait Pattern of walking

Orthotics Supports, splints, or braces used for correction and alignment

Pedorthist Professionals who design, fit, and modify shoes and orthotic devices

PODIATRIST

- Treat common foot problems
- Set fractures and sprains
- Fit for orthotics
- Detect the early stages of disease that exhibit early warning signs in the feet such as arthritis, diabetes, and cardiovascular disease

FOOT CONDITIONS & DISORDERS

Bunions	Large toe angles in toward other toes, causing bump
Calluses	Thickening or build up of skin due to pressure or friction
Flatfoot	Condition in which one or more of the foot arches have flattened out
Hammertoe	Bending of one or more joints in the toes
Neuroma	Overgrowth of nerves around a bone, causing irritation and swelling
Onychocryptosis	Ingrown toenail
Onychomycosis	Fungal infection, causing brittle, thick, and discolored nails
Plantar Fasciitis	Inflammation of the ligament that connects the heel to the toes

Psychiatry

PSYCHIATRY	The study and diagnosis of mental illness
PSYCHIATRIST	Physician specializing in the diagnosis and treatment of mental illness

KEY TERMS

Cognition	Processing thoughts and information
Delirium	Confusion in thoughts and perceptions
Delusion	False personal belief held with great conviction that cannot be changed by reasoning
Dysphoria	State of sadness, restlessness, and irritability
Euphoria	State of intense happiness
Mania	Abnormally elevated state or mood
Neurosis	Repressed conflicts that result in anxiety and fear
Paranoia	Thoughts characterized by excessive fear and anxiety
Phobia	Fear of situations, activities, and things
Psychosis	Delusions, hallucinations, and breaks from reality
Schizophrenic	Cannot distinguish between what is real and what is not real

FUNCTIONAL & ORGANIC DISEASE

Functional Disease
- Physical disorder with no observable change or loss of tissue
- Believed to be psychological in nature

Organic Disease
- Condition in which changes have been observed and destruction of tissue has occurred
- Symptoms can be measured

PSYCHIATISTS AND PSYCHOLOGISTS

Psychiatrists
- Medical Doctor
- Prescribes drugs and electroconvulsive therapy
- Areas of specialization include:
    - Child Psychiatry: Children and adolescents
    - Forensic Psychiatry: Legal aspects
    - Psychoanalysis   Emotions and conflicts
    - Psychopharmacology: Actions and effects of drugs

Psychologists
- Non-medical professional with a doctorate in psychology/counseling
- Do not prescribe drugs or electroconvulsive therapy
- Areas of specialization include:
    - Clinical: Counseling and testing
    - Experimental: Laboratory tests and experiments
    - Social: Social behavior and interaction

PSYCHIATRIC DISORDERS

- Anxiety
- Behavior
- Delirium
- Dementia
- Developmental
- Mood
- Personality
- Schizophrenic
- Sexual and Gender
- Substance

PSYCHIATRIC THERAPIES

Drug Therapy	Incorporates the use of different types of drugs to treat psychiatric disorders
Electroconvulsive Therapy	Incorporates the use of electrical current to produce changes in brainwave patterns
Family Therapy	Treating the entire family to resolve and understand conflicts and problems
Group Therapy	Interacting with others with similar problems in a group setting
Hypnosis Therapy	Being put in a trance or state of altered consciousness
Play Therapy	Incorporates the use of toys to express feelings and conflicts
Psychotherapy	Focuses on the exploration of inner conflicts and disorders

Pulmonology

PULMONOLOGY	The study and treatment of lung diseases and disorders
PULMONOLOGIST	Physician specializing in the diagnosis and treatment of lung diseases and disorders

KEY TERMS

Inhaler	Portable, handheld device that administers a measured amount of medication as a spray directly into the mouth, or as a powder that is inhaled
Nebulizer	Electric or battery-operated machine that administers medication by way of a fine mist that is inhaled using a mouthpiece or mask
Spirometer	Instrument that measures the volume and rate of air passing in and out of the lungs

RESPIRATION

External Respiration
- Exchange of oxygen and carbon dioxide that occurs between the environment and the lungs
- Process of inhaling and exhaling air; breathing

Internal Respiration
- Exchange of oxygen and carbon dioxide that occurs in the body tissues
- Cells absorb oxygen and release carbon dioxide

PULMONARY CONDITIONS & DISORDERS

Apnea	Absence of breathing
Asthma	Inflammation of the airway passages making breathing difficult
Bradypnea	Slow breathing rate
Chronic Bronchitis	Chronic cough with production of mucus and inflamed airways
Chronic Obstructive Pulmonary Disease (COPD)	Any disorder that consistently obstructs airflow to the lungs
Cystic Fibrosis (CF)	Genetic disease characterized by the excessive production of mucous
Dyspnea	Labored or difficulty breathing; shortness of breath
Emphysema	Abnormal accumulation of air sacs in the lungs
Hyperventilation	Abnormally fast and deep breathing
Pneumonia	Infection of one or both of the lungs
Pulmonary Edema	Build up of fluid in the lungs
Tachypnea	Rapid breathing
Tuberculosis	Bacterial infection of the lungs

PULMONARY TESTS

Arterial Blood Gases (ABG)	Lab test to detect lung diseases
Blood Gas Diffusion Test	Measures how well oxygen and carbon dioxide are absorbed into the blood
Bronchoscopy	Examination of the airways using a viewing tube
Pulmonary Function Tests (PFT)	Group of tests that evaluate lung function
Spirometry Test	Measures how efficiently air moves in and out of the lungs
Thoracoscopy	Examination of the surface of the lungs using a flexible viewing tube

Radiology

Radiology	The use of radiation and imaging technology to diagnose and treat disease
Radiologist	Physician who uses radiation and imaging technology to diagnose and treat disease

KEY TERMS

CT Scan Computed Tomography; more detailed test than an x-ray, which uses a combination of x-ray and computer technology to produce cross-sectional images (slices) to focus on precise sections of the body

Fluoroscopy Test using a continuous x-ray image to produce moving (movie-like) images of the body

MRI Magnetic Resonance Imaging; testing using a combination of magnets, radio frequencies, and computer technology to produce detailed images of internal organs and body structures

Ultrasound Technique using high-frequency sound waves to create images of internal organs

X-Ray Radiography; diagnostic test that uses invisible electromagnetic beams to produce images of the internal tissues, bones, and organs

PROCEDURES/STUDIES

Contrast Contrast media, such as iodine-based substances and barium, are administered to improve the visualization of organs and tissues

Tracer Radionuclides attach to chemicals and are followed as they travel through the body

Ventilation-Perfusion Radiopharmaceuticals are inhaled (ventilation) and injected intravenously (perfusion); imaging follows their passage through the respiratory track

RADIOGRAPHIC TESTING

DIAGNOSTIC	The use of various radiology techniques, X-ray, CT scan, MRI, ultrasound, and fluoroscopy to diagnose a medical condition
INTERVENTIONAL	A specialty area of radiology that uses various techniques such as x-ray, CT scans, MRI, ultrasound, and tools (wires and tubes) to perform procedures through a very small opening in the skin
NUCLEAR	Testing incorporating the use of x-ray and small amounts of radioactive substances. Patient digests a radiopharmaceutical substance, or it is injected into the vein with a small amount of radioactive material
RADIATION	The use of high-energy waves to damage cancer cells and stop them from growing and dividing

Rheumatology

Rheumatology	The study and nonsurgical treatment of the joints and connective tissue
Rheumatologist	Physician specializing in the diagnosis, treatment, and management of joint pain, inflammation and muscle soreness and stiffness

KEY TERMS

Arthritis   Inflammation in the joint

Degenerative Progressive impairment

Inflammation Response of the tissue to injury

INFLAMMATION

Inflammation is characterized by:

- Redness
- Joint pain and stiffness
- Swollen joint that is warm to the touch
- Loss of joint function

Inflammation may be associated with flu-like symptoms:

- Fever
- Headache
- Chills
- Fatigue
- Loss of appetite

Results of Inflammation:

- Irritation and swelling of the joint lining
- Wearing down of cartilage

ARTHRITIS

Inflammation of the joints causing pain, stiffness, swelling, tenderness, redness, warmth and difficulty with movement

- Common causes:
  - Age
  - Autoimmune disease
  - Infection
  - Occupational hazards
  - Previous injury
  - Weight

- There are over 100 types of arthritis including:
  - Osteoarthritis: Degenerative disease with loss of cartilage
  - Rheumatoid: Chronic, inflammatory disease characterized by painful joints
  - Juvenile Rheumatoid: Rheumatoid arthritis occurring in children and adolescents
  - Gout: Inflammation of the joints caused by excessive uric acid
  - Ankylosing Spondylitis: Inflammation of the joints between the spine and the pelvis
  - Scleroderma: Connective tissue disease that hardens and stiffens skin

RHEUMATOID CONDITIONS & DISORDERS

Fibromyalgia   Chronic, musculoskeletal disease that causes pain and fatigue

Lupus   Chronic, inflammatory disease that attacks the healthy tissues and organs

Lyme Disease   Bacterial infection and disease characterized by severe fatigue, fever, headache and muscle and joint pain

RHEUMATOLOGY LAB TESTS

Antinuclear Antibody (ANA)   Determines presence of autoimmune disease

Erythrocyte Sedimentation Rate (ESR)   Determines the cause of inflammation

Rheumatoid Factor (RF)   Determines presence of the RF antibody

Urology

Urology	The study and treatment of the urinary tract in men and women and the reproductive tract in men
Urologist	Physician specializing in diseases and disorders of the urinary tract in men and women and the reproductive tract in men

KEY TERMS

Urinalysis	Collection of urine for testing
• Clean Catch	Urine is collected mid stream to avoid contamination
• Random	Urine is collected at any time
• Timed	Urine is collected over time
• Urine Dipstick	Testing strip is placed in urine specimen that identifies the presence of disease

URINARY SYSTEM	
Kidneys	Filter waste products from the blood and disposes of them by creating urine; regulates the amount of water in the body
Ureters	Long tubes that carry urine form the kidneys to the urinary bladder
Urinary Bladder	Muscular sac that holds urine until it is ready to be excreted
Urethra	Tube from the bladder to the external opening of the body that allows for the passage of urine

UROLOGICAL CONDITIONS & DISORDERS

Benign Prostatic Hyperplasia (BPH) Enlarged prostate gland

Dysuria Painful passing of urine

Hematuria Blood in urine

Prostatitis Inflammation of the prostate

Urge Incontinence Overactive bladder; sudden, strong need to urinate

Urinary Incontinence Loss of bladder control; involuntary loss of urine

Urinary Retention Inability to urinate

Urinary Tract Infection (UTI) Infection of the kidneys and bladder

UROLOGICAL TESTS AND PROCEDURES

Blood Urea Nitrogen (BUN) Blood test that measures the level of the waste product urea in the blood

Creatinine Clearance Test that measures the rate of the kidneys in removing the waste product creatinine from the blood

Cystography Diagnostic test that uses contrast medium to examine the urinary bladder

Cystometry Diagnostic test used to evaluate the filling and emptying rates of the bladder

Cystoscopy Test using a lighted, flexible viewing tube to examine the urinary tract

Prostate Specific Antigen (PSA) Test that measures the amount of the prostate specific antigen protein in the blood

Urinalysis Test that determines the presence of abnormal elements in the urine

Uroflowmetry Test that calculates the flow of urine over a period of time

Wound Care

WOUND CARE	Care and treatment of chronic wounds
WOUND CARE SPECIALIST	Practitioner specializing in the treatment of chronic and non-healing wounds

KEY TERMS

Abrasion	Wound where the top layer of skin is torn off
Avulsion	Wound where tissue is completely torn from body
Contusion	Bruise; blunt force injury
Debridement	Surgical removal of tissue and metabolic waste
Incision	Wound made from a sharp razor-like object
Laceration	Jagged-edge cut
Puncture	Wound made from a sharp, pointed object

CHRONIC WOUNDS

Wounds that do not begin to heal within four weeks, or wounds that have not healed in twelve weeks

• Diabetic ulcers	Break down of the skin on the foot
• Pressure ulcers	Bedsore, result of an immobilizing disorder
• Venous ulcers	Open wound due to an inadequate blood supply

STAGES OF HEALING	
Inflammation	Bleeding, redness, swelling and clot formation
Proliferation	Formation of new blood vessels
Reconstruction	Collagen production, tissue growth
Epithelialization	Growth of new skin

MY KEY NOTES

Credits & Acknowledgements

American Cancer Association
http://www.cancer.org

American Heart Association
http://www.heart.org

American Medical Association
http://www.ama-assn.org

BlueCross BlueShield Association
http://www.bcbs.com

Centers for Disease Control and Prevention
http://www.cdc.gov

Centers for Medicare & Medicaid Services
http://www.cms.gov

Department of Veterans Affairs
http://www.va.gov

Drug Enforcement Administration
http://www.justice.gov/dea

Internal Revenue Service
http://www.irs.gov

Joint Commission
http://www.jointcommission.org

Mayo Clinic
http://www.mayoclinic.com

National Library of Medicine
http://www.nlm.nih.gov

Occupational Safety and Health Administration
http://www.osha.org

Tricare
http://www.tricare.mil

United States Department of Health and Human Services
http://www.hhs.gov

United States Department of Justice
http://www.justice.gov

United States Department of Labor
http://www.dol.gov

United States Department of the Treasury
http://www.treasury.gov

Acronyms

ADHD	Attention Deficit Hyperactivity Disorder
AFIB	Atrial Fibrillation
AIDS	Acquired Immunodeficiency Syndrome
AMA	American Medical Association
ANA	Antinuclear Antibody
AND	Associate Degree in Nursing
APN	Advanced Practice Nurse
BMP	Basic Metabolic Panel
BP	Blood Pressure
BPH	Benign Prostatic Hypertrophy
BSN	Bachelor of Science Nursing
BUN	Blood Urea Nitrogen
CAD	Coronary Artery Disease
CAT	Computerized Axial Tomography
CBC	Complete Blood Count
CC	Chief Complaint
CF	Cystic Fibrosis
CHAMPUS	Civilian Health and Medical Program of the Uniformed Services
CHAMPVA	Civilian Health and Medical Program of Veterans Affairs
CHD	Coronary Heart Disease
CHF	Congestive Heart failure
CHIP	Children's Health Insurance Program
CKD	Chronic Kidney Disease
CMS	Centers for Medicare and Medicaid Services
CNS	Central Nervous System
COB	Coordination of Benefits
COPD	Chronic Obstructive Pulmonary Disease
CPR	Cardiopulmonary Resuscitation
CPT-4	Current Procedural Terminology Fourth Edition
CRF	Chronic Renal Failure
CSF	Cerebrospinal Fluid
CT	Computed Tomography
CVA	Cerebrovascular Accident
CXR	Chest X-ray
DJD	Degenerative Joint Disease
DM	Diabetes Mellitus
DO	Doctor of Osteopathy
DTP	Diphtheria, Tetanus, Pertussis
DVT	Deep Vein Thrombosis
DX	Diagnosis
ECHO	Echocardiogram
EEG	Electroencephalogram
EKG	Electrocardiogram
ELISA	Enzyme-linked Immunosorbent Assay
EMG	Electromyography
EMR	Electronic Medical Record

EMTALA	Emergency Medical Treatment and Active Labor Act
ENG	Electronystagmography
ENT	Ears, Nose, Throat
EOB	Explanation of Benefits
EPO	Exclusive Provider Organization
ESR	Erythrocyte Sedimentation Rate
ESRD	End-stage Renal Disease
FEHB	Federal Employees Health Benefits
FFS	Fee For Service
FSA	Flexible Spending Account
FSH	Follicle Stimulating Hormone
GERD	Gastroesophageal Reflux Disease
GFR	Glomerular Filtration Rate
GI	Gastrointestinal
GU	Genitourinary
GYN	Gynecology
HAV	Hepatitis A Virus
HBV	Hepatitis B Virus
HCPCS	Healthcare Common Procedure Coding System
HCT	Hematocrit
HCV	Hepatitis C Virus
HDL	High Density Lipoprotein
HGB	Hemoglobin
HIPAA	Health Insurance Portability and Accountability Act
HIV	Human Immunodeficiency Virus
HMO	Health Maintenance Organization
HPV	Human Papilloma Virus
HRT	Hormone Replacement Therapy
HSA	Health Savings Account
HTN	Hypertension
IBD	Inflammatory Bowel Disease
IBS	Irritable Bowel Syndrome
ICD-10 CM	International Classification of Diseases Tenth Revision, Clinical Modification
ICD-9 CM	International Classification of Diseases Ninth Revision, Clinical Modification
IDDM	Insulin-Dependent Diabetes Mellitus
IHS	Indian Health Service
IM	Intramuscular
IV	Intravenous
JC	Joint Commission
JCAHO	Joint Commission on the Accreditation of Healthcare Organizations
LDL	Low Density Lipoprotein
LOC	Level of Care
LPN	Licensed Practical Nurse
LVN	Licensed Vocational Nurse
MA	Medical Assistant
MC	Managed Care

MCO	Managed Care Organization
MD	Medical Doctor
MI	Myocardial Infarction
MMR	Measles, Mumps, Rubella
MRI	Magnetic Resonance Imaging
MRSA	Methicillin-Resistant Staphylococcus Aureus
MS	Multiple Sclerosis
MSA	Medical Savings Account
MVA	Motor Vehicle Accident
NCV	Nerve Conduction Velocity
NIDDM	Non-Insulin Dependent Diabetes Mellitus
NKA	No Known Allergies
NKDA	No Known Drug Allergies
NP	Nurse Practitioner
NPI	National Provider Identifier
NPP	Notice of Privacy Practices
OB	Obstetrics
OSHA	Occupational Safety and Health Administration
OT	Occupational Therapy
PA	Physician Assistant
PAD	Peripheral Artery Disease
PCP	Primary Care Provider
PET	Positron Emission Tomography
PFT	Pulmonary Function Test
PHI	Protected Health Information
PID	Pelvic Inflammatory Disease
PKD	Polycystic Kidney Disease
PMS	Premenstrual Syndrome
PNS	Peripheral Nervous System
POS	Point of Service
PPO	Preferred Provider Organization
PSA	Prostate Specific Antigen
PUD	Peptic Ulcer Disease
RA	Rheumatoid Arthritis
RAST	Radioallergosorbent Test
RBC	Red Blood Cell
RF	Rheumatoid Factor
RN	Registered Nurse
SOB	Shortness of Breathe
STD	Sexually Transmitted Disease
TB	Tuberculosis
TIA	Transient Ischemic Attack
TSH	Thyroid Stimulating Hormone
UA	Urinalysis
URI	Upper Respiratory Infection
UTI	Urinary Tract Infection
WBC	White Blood Cell
WC	Workers' Compensation
WHO	World Health Organization

Index

A

abrasion, 119
absorption, 80
acne, 77
acquired immune deficiency
acquired immunity, 66
active chart, 35
acuity, 69
acute pain, 102
administrative staff, 15, 18
advance beneficiary notice (ABN), 54
advanced practice nurse (APN), 16
affiliated provider, 55
age-related care, 19
age-related specialties, 65
    syndrome (AIDS), 86-87
AIDS. *See* acquired immune
    deficiency syndrome
allergen(s), 66, 67
allergic response, 66, 67
allergist, 66
allergy tests, 67
allergy, 66-67, 101
Alzheimer's disease, 93
ambulatory care, 19
American Cancer Society ABCD
    Rule, 77
American Medical Association
    (AMA), 43
analgesics, 104
anaphylaxis, 66
anemia
    autoimmune disease, 68
    medical coding, 46
    types, 85
anesthetics, 104
aneurysm, 71
angina, 71
ankylosing spondylitis, 116
antibiotics, 104
antibody, 66
anticoagulants, 104
antidepressants, 104
antigen, 66, 68

antihistamine, 66, 104
antiplatelet, 104
antivirals, 104
apnea, 112
appointment scheduling, 22-23
appointment types, 22
arrhythmia, 73
arteriosclerosis, 73
arthritis,
    autoimmune disease, 68
    definition, 116
    physical therapy, 107
    podiatry, 108
    types, 116
arthrography, 100
arthroplasty, 100
arthroscopy, 100
asthma, 112
astigmatism, 98
atrial fibrillation (AFIB), 73
audiogram, 69
audiologist, 21, 69
audiology, 21, 69
audiometer, 69
audiometry, 69
auditory canal, 69, 70
auditory liquids, 69, 70
auditory nerve fibers, 69, 70
auditory receptor cells, 69, 70
auscultation, 71
authorization
    definition, 8
    form, 35
    HIPAA privacy rule, 12
    patient rights, 11
    referral, 54
    to release information, 36
autism, 93
autoimmune disease, 68, 116
avulsion, 119

B

barium
    contrast studies, 113

definition, 80
  enema, 83
  swallow, 83
basic metabolic panel (BMP), 89
beneficiary, 55
benign, 95
benign prostatic hyperplasia (BPH),
  118
bile, 80
biller
  administrative staff, 15, 18
  job process, 25
  roles in reimbursement, 38
biopsy
  collection, 88
  definition, 88
  liver, 83
birthday rule, 63
blepharitis, 98
blood, 84–85
  leukemia, 96
  specimen collection, 88
  transmission of disease, 87
blood enzyme test, 89
blood gas diffusion test, 112
blood organs, 84
blood pressure (BP)
  abbreviation, 32
  adrenal gland, 79
  definition, 72
  hypertension, 73
  hypotension, 71
  kidneys, 90
  nervous system, 92
blood sugar, 78
blood system, 85
blood tests,
  allergy, 67
  antinuclear antibody (ANA), 116
  arterial blood gases (ABG),
  basic metabolic panel (BMP), 89
  blood enzymes, 89
  blood gas diffusion, 112
  blood urea nitrogen (BUN), 118
  complete blood count (CBC), 89
  ELISA, 67
  erythrocyte sedimentation
  rate (ESR), 116

fecal occult blood test (FOBT), 83
  glomerular filtration rate (GMR),
  91
  lipid panel, 89
  prostate specific antigen (PSA),
  118
  RAST, 67
  rheumatoid factor (RF), 116
  routine, 89
blood urea nitrogen (BUN), 118
blood vessels, 71, 72, 73
body language, 3
bone density, 100
bone scan, 100
bones, 99–100
bradycardia
  definition, 71
  medical terminology, 34
bradypnea, 112
brain, 21, 92, 93
brain stem, 93
brand name drug, 103
bronchoscopy, 112
bunions, 108
bursitis, 100

C

calluses, 108
cancer, 21, 95–96
  carcinoma, 96
  leukemia, 96
  lymphoma, 96
  sarcoma, 96
  skin, 77
capitation, 54
carcinogenesis, 95
carcinoma, 95, 96
cardiac surgeon, 71
cardiologist, 21, 71
cardiology, 21, 71–73
carpal tunnel, 100
carpals, 100
carrier, 55
cartilage, 99, 100
cataract, 98
cavitation, 74
celiac disease, 82
cells, 84

cellulitis, 77
Centers for Medicare and Medicaid
    Services (CMS), 43, 60
central nervous system (CNS), 92
cerebellum, 93
cerebral palsy (CP), 93
cerebrospinal fluid analysis (CFS), 93
cerebrovascular accident (CVA), 73
cerebrum, 93
certification, 17
cerumen, 69
cervical, 74, 75
CHAMPUS. *See* Civilian Health and
    Medical Program of the
    Uniformed Services
CHAMPVA. *See* Civilian Health and
    Medical Services of Veterans
    Affairs
charge entry, 38
chart(s)
    active, 35
    closed, 35
    delinquent, 35
    electronic medical record, 28
    hybrid, 28
    inactive, 35
    incomplete, 35
    organization, 28
    paper, 28
    TABS, 28, 29
chemical name drug, 103
child psychology, 109
Children's Health Insurance
    Program(CHIP), 53, 62
CHIP. *See* Children's Health
    Insurance Program
chiropractic medicine, 74–75
chiropractor, 74, 75
chronic bronchitis, 112
chronic kidney disease (CKD), 91
chronic obstructive pulmonary
    disease(COPD), 112
chronic pain, 102
chronic renal failure (CRF), 91
chronic wounds, 119
circulatory system, 72
cirrhosis, 82
Civilian Health and Medical
    Program of Uniformed Service

(CHAMPUS), 62
Civilian Health and Medical
    Program of Veterans Affairs
    (CHAMPVA), 62
claimant, 55
claims, 38
clavicle, 100
clinical psychology, 109
clinical staff, 15, 16–17
closed chart, 35
CMS. *See* Centers for Medicare and
    Medicaid Services
COBRA. *See* Consolidated Omnibus
    Reconciliation Act
COBRA law, 13
coccyx, 74
cochlea, 69, 70
cochlear implants, 70
coder, 18
coding
    assigning, 50
    coding for coverage, 51
    compliance, 51
    CPT-4, 43, 48-49
    E codes, 47
    E&M codes, 48-49
    G codes, 49
    guidelines, 50
    HCPCS, 43
    ICD-10 CM, 47
    ICD-9 CM, 43, 44-47
    highest degree of specialization,
    46
    illegal billing practices, 51
    J codes, 49
    medical necessity rule, 51
    modifiers, 50
    reimbursement, 38
    significance of, 44
    unbundling, 51
    up-coding, 51
    V codes, 46
cognition, 109
coinsurance, 54
collagen, 76
colonoscopy, 83
color blindness, 98
commercial insurance, 53, 57–59
complete blood count (CBC), 89

complete chart, 35
complete fracture, 99
compound fracture, 99
computed tomography, 113
confidentiality, 8, 11, 35
congestive heart failure (CHF), 73
conjunctivitis, 98
consent
    expressed, 8
    implied, 8
    informed, 8, 11, 36
Consolidated Omnibus
    Reconciliation Act (COBRA), 13,
    54
constipation, 82
continuing care, 20
contrast studies, 113
controlled substance act, 105
cornea, 97
corneal abrasion, 98
corneal laceration, 98
coronary artery disease (CAD), 73
covered entity, 9
CPT-4. *See* Current Procedural
    Terminology Fourth Edition
cranium, 100
creatinine clearance, 118
Crohn's disease, 82
CT scan, 113
culture, 88
Current Procedural Terminology
    4th Edition (CPT-4), 43, 48–49
    G codes, 49
    J codes, 49
customer service, 1–5
    body language, 3
    customer service 5/10 rule, 3
    difficult people, 4
    listening, 3
cystic fibrosis (CF), 112
cystography, 118
cystolithiasis, 91
cystometry, 118
cystoscopy, 118

D
debridement, 119
decedent, 55
deductible, 54

deep vein thrombosis (DVT), 73
defecation, 80, 81
degenerative, 115
deglutition, 80, 81
delinquent chart, 35
delirium, 109
delusion, 109
demographic. *See* patient
    demographics
dependent, 55
dermatitis, 77
dermatologist, 21, 76
dermatology, 21, 76–77
detached retina, 98
diabetes, 79
diabetic ulcers, 119
diagnosis (DX), 22
diagnostic testing, 114
dialysis, 91
diarrhea, 82
difficult people, 4
digestion, 80
dilation test, 98
disc, 99
disclosure, 8, 10, 11, 12
dislocation, 74
diverticulitis, 82
Doctor of osteopathy (DO), 16
documentation, 31–32
drug categories, 104
drug therapy, 110
dysphagia, 82, 101
dysphoria, 109
dysplasia, 95
dyspnea, 112
dysuria, 117

E
E codes, 47
ear, 101
echocardiogram (ECHO), 73
echocardiogram stress test, 73
ectopic pregnancy, 94
eczema, 77
elastin, 76
electrocardiogram (EKG), 73
electrocardiogram stress test, 73
electroconvulsive therapy, 110
electroencephalogram (EEG), 93

electromyography (EMG), 93
electronic medical records (EMR), 28, 30
electronystagmography (ENG), 93
elimination, 80
ELISA test. *See* Enzyme-Linked Immunosorbent Assay
E&M codes. *See* evaluation and management codes
embolism, 71
emergency care, 19
Emergency Medical Treatment and Active Labor Act (EMTALA), 13
emphysema, 112
EMR. *See* Electronic Medical Records
EMTALA. *See* Emergency Treatment and Active Labor Act
encounter form, 22, 25, 27, 38, 51
end stage renal disease (ESRD), 91
endocrine glands, 79
endocrine laboratory tests, 79
endocrine system, 78
endocrinologist, 21, 78
endocrinology, 21, 78–79
endometriosis, 94
endoscopy, 83
   arthroscopy, 100
   bronchoscopy, 112
   colonoscopy, 83
   cystoscopy, 118
   enteroscopy, 83
   esophagoscopy, 83
   gastroscopy, 83
   laparoscopy, 83
   sigmoidoscopy, 83
   thoracoscopy, 112
   upper endoscopy, 83
enrollee, 55
enteroscopy, 83
Enzyme-Linked Immunosorbent Assay (ELISA), 67
enzymes, 80
epidemic, 86
epiglottis, 101
epilepsy, 93
epithelialization, 119
EPO. *See* exclusive provider organization
erythrocytes, 84

esophagitis, 82
esophagoscopy, 83
established patient, 25
estrogen, 94
euphoria, 109
evaluation and management (E&M) code(s), 48, 49, 51
Exclusive provider organization (EPO), 57, 58
excretion, 90
expectorate, 88
experimental psychology, 109
expressed consent, 8
external respiration, 111
eye, 97–98
eye conditions and disorders, 98
eye tests, 98

F

family medicine, 19
family therapy, 110
fecal occult blood test, 83
Federal Employees Health Benefits (FEHB), 53, 62
fee for service plans (FFS), 53, 59
fee schedule, 8
FEHB. *See* Federal Employees Health Benefits
femur, 100
FFS. *See* fee for service plans
fibrocystic breast, 94
fibroids, 94
fibromyalgia, 116
fibula, 100
filing systems, 39
filtration, 90
flatfoot, 108
flexible spending account (FSA), 59
fluoroscopy, 113
foot conditions and disorders, 108
forensic psychology, 109
formulary drug, 103
fracture, 99
front office fundamentals, 15
front office staff, 18
FSA. *See* flexible spending account
functional disease, 109
fungal infection, 86

G

G codes, 49
gait, 108
gastric, 80
gastroenterologist, 80
gastroenterology, 80–83
gastroesophageal reflux
    disease (GERD), 82
gastroscopy, 83
gatekeeper, 55
generic name drug, 103
geriatric medicine, 19
gestational diabetes, 79
gland(s)
    definition, 78
    endocrine, 79
    sebaceous, 76
    sweat, 76
glaucoma test, 98
glaucoma, 98
glomerular filtration rate (GFR), 91
glucose, 78
gout, 116
government programs, 53, 60-62
granulation, 119
group therapy, 110
guarantor, 55
gynecologist, 21, 94
gynecology, 21, 94

H

hammertoe, 108
HCPCS. *See* Healthcare Common
    Procedure Coding System
health care environments, 19
health insurance, 53
Health Insurance Portability and
    Accountability Act (HIPAA), 7, 8,
    9, 12
Health maintenance organization
    (HMO), 57
Health savings account (HSA), 53, 59
Healthcare Common Procedure
    Coding System (HCPCS), 43
hearing aids, 70
hematocrit, 84
hematologist, 21, 84
hematology, 21, 84–85
hematuria, 117

hemodialysis, 91
hemoglobin, 84
hemophilia, 85
hepatitis (HEP), 82
HIPAA. *See* Health Insurance
    Portability and Accountability
    Act
HIPAA Privacy Rule, 8, 12
HIPAA Security Rule, 8
histamine, 66
HIV. *See* human immunodeficiency
    virus
HMO. *See* health maintenance
    organization
holter monitor, 73
hormone, 78
hospice care, 20
Human immunodeficiency virus
    (HIV), 86, 87
humorous, 100
hybrid chart, 28
hyperglycemia, 79
hyperlipidemia, 79
hyperopia, 98
hyperplasia, 95
hypertension, (HTN) 73
hyperthyroidism, 79
hyperventilation, 112
hypnosis therapy, 110
hypoglycemia, 79
hypolipidemia, 79
hypotension, 71
hypothalamus, 93
hypothyroidism,79

I

ICD-9 CM. *See* International
    Classification of Disease Ninth
    Edition Clinical Modification
ICD-10 CM. *See* International
    Classification of Diseases Tenth
    Revision, Clinical Modification
IHS. *See* Indian Health Service
illegal billing practices, 50
immune response, 66
immune system, 68
immunity, 66
immunologist, 66
immunology, 66, 68

impetigo, 77
implied consent, 8
in situ, 95
inactive chart, 35
incision, 119
incomplete chart, 35
incomplete fracture, 99
indemnity insurance, 59
Indian Health Service (IHS), 53, 62
infarction, 71
infection(s), 86
infectious disease specialist, 86
infectious disease, 86–87
infertility, 94
inflammation, 115, 119
inflammatory bowel disease (IBD), 82
inflammatory response, 66
informed consent, 9, 11, 36
inhalation,
inhaler, 111
insulin, 78
insured, 55
insurer, 55
internal medicine, 19
internal respiration, 111
International Classification of Diseases Ninth Revision, Clinical Modification (ICD-9 CM), 43, 44–47
  E codes, 47
  tabular index, 45
  V codes, 46
International Classification of Diseases Tenth Revision, Clinical Modification (ICD-10 CM), 43
interventional testing, 114
iris, 97
iron deficiency anemia, 85
irritable bowel syndrome (IBS), 82
ischemia, 71

J

J codes, 4
JC. *See* Joint Commission
JCAHCO. *See* Joint Commission on Organizations (JC), 12
joint, 99
Joint Commission on the

Accreditation of Health Care Organizations, 12

K

kidneys, 21, 78, 90, 91, 96, 117, 118

L

laboratory, 88–90
  blood tests, 89
  laboratory technician, 17
  specimen collection, 88
laceration, 119
laparoscopy, 83
laryngitis, 101
larynx, 101
lens, 97
leukemia, 95, 96
leukocytes, 84
level of care (LOC), 49
licensed practical nurse (LPN), 17
licensed vocational nurse (LVN), 17
licensure, 17
ligament, 99, 100
lipid panel, 89
listening, 3
liver biopsy, 83
lower gastrointestinal tract, 81
lumbar, 74
lupus, 116
luxation, 74
Lyme disease, 86, 116
lymph, 71
lymphatic system, 72
lymphedema, 73
lymphoma, 95, 96

M

macula, 97
macular degeneration, 98
magnetic resonance reasoning (MRI), 113
major medical insurance, 59
malignant, 95
managed care organization(s) (MCO), 53, 57–58
mandible, 100
mania, 109
manipulation, 74
mastication, 80, 81

9, 10, 11, 12, 36, 37
protocol, 35
provider, 56
psoriasis, 77
psychiatric therapies, 110
psychiatrist, 21, 109-110
psychiatry, 21, 109–110
psychoanalysis, 109
psychologist, 109-110
psychology, 109-110
psychopharmacology, 109
public insurance, 53, 60–62
pulmonologist, 21, 111
pulmonology, 21, 111–112
puncture, 119
pupil, 97

R

radiation testing, 114
radiographic testing, 114
radiologist, 113
radiology, 113–114
   procedures, 113
   testing, 114
radius, 100
RAST test, 67
reabsorption, 90
reconstruction, 119
rectal, 103
referral, 54
refraction test, 98
registered nurse (RN), 16
registration, 17
reimbursement, 12, 15, 25, 28, 31, 38,
   44, 50, 51
rejected claim, 38
respiration, 111
respite care, 20
responsible party, 56
restorative care, 20
retina, 97
rheumatologist, 21, 115
rheumatology, 21, 115–116
rhinitis, 101
routes of administering medicine,
   103

S

sacral, 74

sarcoma, 95
scapula, 100
schizophrenic, 109
sclera, 97
scleroderma, 11
scoliosis, 100
sebaceous glands, 76
seborrhea, 77
second surgical opinion, 54
secondary care, 19
secretion, 90
sedatives, 104
sepsis, 85
sickle cell anemia, 85
sigmoidoscopy, 83
simple fracture, 99
sinus rhythm, 71
sinusitis, 101
skin, 76
skin cancer, 77
skin tests,
   intradermal, 67
   patch, 67
   prick, 67
slit lamp exam, 98
SOAP documentation, 32
social psychology, 109
somatic pain, 102
sound, 70
specialist, 56
specimen, 88
specimen collection
   expectorate, 88
   needle biopsy, 88
   open biopsy, 88
   stool sample, 88
   swab, 88
   urinalysis, 88
   venipuncture, 88
spine, 75
spirometer, 111
spirometry test, 112
sprain, 99, 100
stages of healing, 119
stenosis, 71
sternum, 100
stimulants, 104
stool sample, 88
strain, 99, 100

sublingual, 103
subluxation, 74
subscriber, 56
surgical specialties, 65
swab, 88
sweat glands, 76

T

U

V

venipuncture, 88
venous ulcers, 119
ventilation-perfusion studies, 113
vertebrae, 99
vertebrate, 99, 100
vertigo, 101viral infection, 86
visceral pain, 102
visual field test, 98
vitamin deficient anemia, 85
vitreous body, 97
Von Willebrand disease, 85

W
World Health Organization (WHO), 43
wound care, 119
wound care specialist, 119

X
x-ray, 113

MY KEY NOTES

MY KEY NOTES

MY KEY NOTES

MY KEY NOTES

MY KEY NOTES

MY KEY NOTES

MY KEY NOTES

MY KEY NOTES

MY KEY NOTES

Made in the USA
San Bernardino, CA
25 May 2013